PEDIATRIC COLLECTIONS
Digital Media

EDITED BY:

Tiffany Munzer, MD, FAAP
Member of AAP Council on Communications and Media Executive Committee
Assistant Professor of Pediatrics; Division of Developmental Behavioral Pediatrics
University of Michigan, Ann Arbor, MI

Jenny Radesky, MD, FAAP
Chair, AAP Council on Communications and Media
Associate Professor of Pediatrics and Division Director
Developmental Behavioral Pediatrics
University of Michigan, Ann Arbor, MI

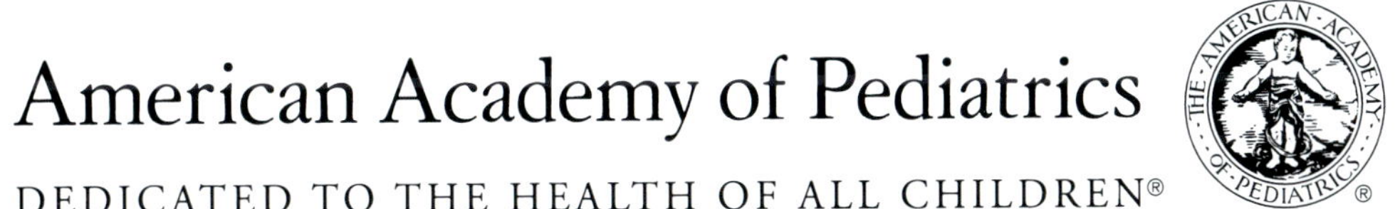
American Academy of Pediatrics

DEDICATED TO THE HEALTH OF ALL CHILDREN®

Published by the American Academy of Pediatrics
345 Park Blvd.
Itasca, IL 60143

Printed in the United States of America

APC043

Print ISBN: 978-1-61002-797-7
eBook ISBN: 978-1-61002-798-4

PEDIATRIC COLLECTIONS

Digital Media

Table of Contents

Digital Media

Part 2: Media Effects

About AAP Pediatric Collections

Pediatric Collections is a series of selected pediatric articles that highlight different facets of information across various AAP publications, including AAP Journals, AAP News, Blog Articles, and eBooks. Each series of collections focuses on specific topics in the field of pediatrics so that you can keep up with best practices, and make an informed response to public health matters, trending news, and current events. Each collection includes previously published content focusing on specific topics and articles selected by AAP editors.

Visit http://collections.aap.org to view online collections that include the most up-to-date AAP content on each subject.

Digital Media

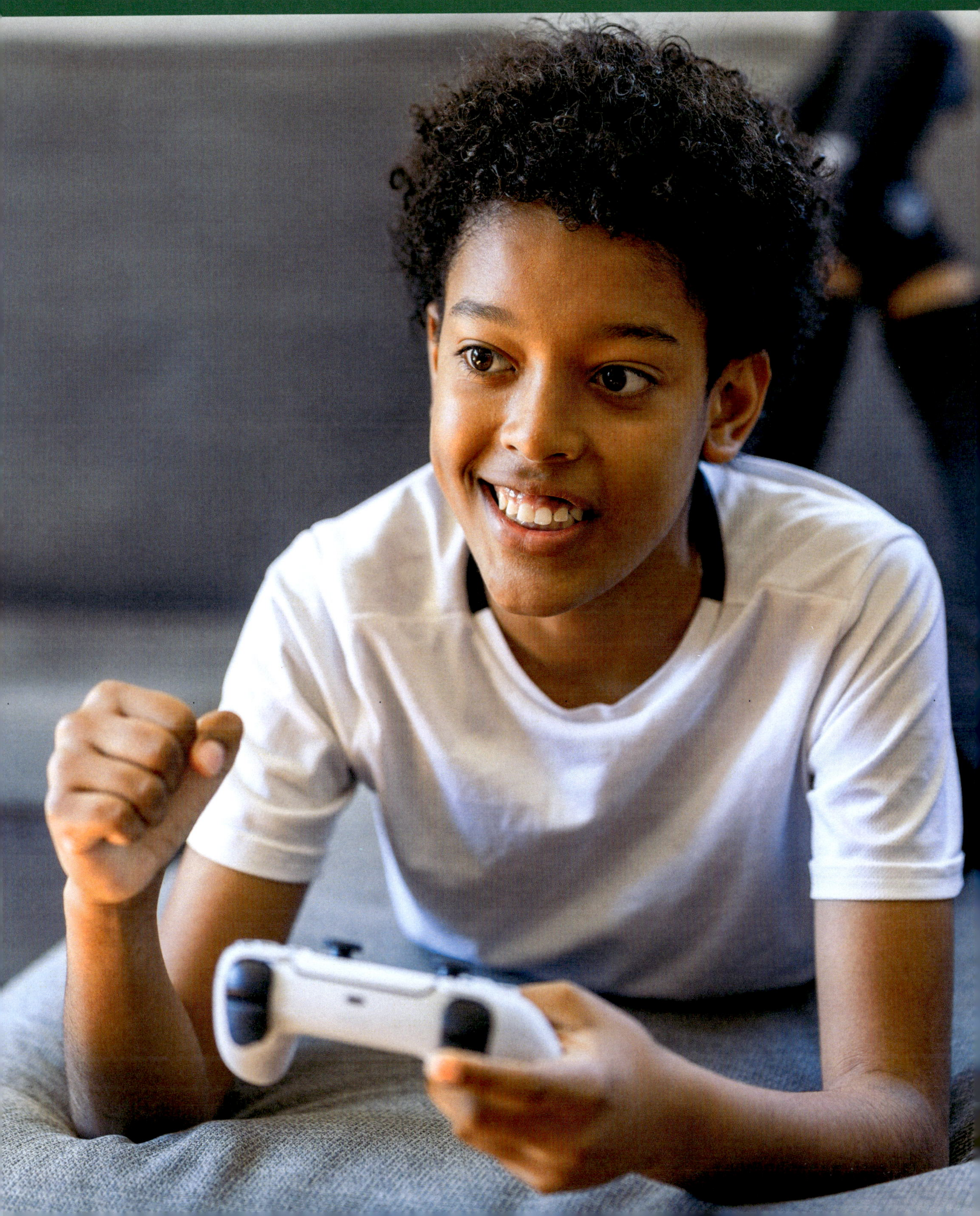

Digital Media
Series Introduction

Tiffany Munzer, MD, FAAP
Member of AAP Council on Communications and Media Executive Committee
Assistant Professor of Pediatrics; Division of Developmental Behavioral Pediatrics
University of Michigan, Ann Arbor, MI

Jenny Radesky, MD, FAAP
Chair, AAP Council on Communications and Media
Associate Professor of Pediatrics and Division Director, Developmental Behavioral Pediatrics
University of Michigan, Ann Arbor, MI

We are pleased to present this collection about digital media and its impact on children's health and well-being. Digital spaces are interwoven into the fabric of children's and families' lives. No longer just the simple concept of "screen time," digital media must be evaluated in the context of physical and social spaces that children occupy, as well as the societal structures that provide or limit children's opportunities. This collection of articles focuses on the ecosystems that shape child and family interactions with digital media, the effects of digital media on children, and the potential that digital media may have in creating opportunities.

This collection is divided into 3 parts—*Part 1: Ecosystems, Part 2: Media Effects, and Part 3: Use of Media as a Tool*—with the goal of highlighting where the science on this topic has been over the past 10 years and where it can go next. Part 1 highlights the importance of transforming the ecosystems that shape children's and families' well-being, so that all children can thrive in both physical and digital spaces. Parts 2 and 3 of this series underscore that the degree to which digital media platforms are or are not designed to be child-centered determines whether they will have a positive or negative impact on children. Therefore, changes and digital media intervention need to occur at a high level, from the top down, to ensure that the digital ecosystem supports families' well-being across the board.

Part 2: Media Effects

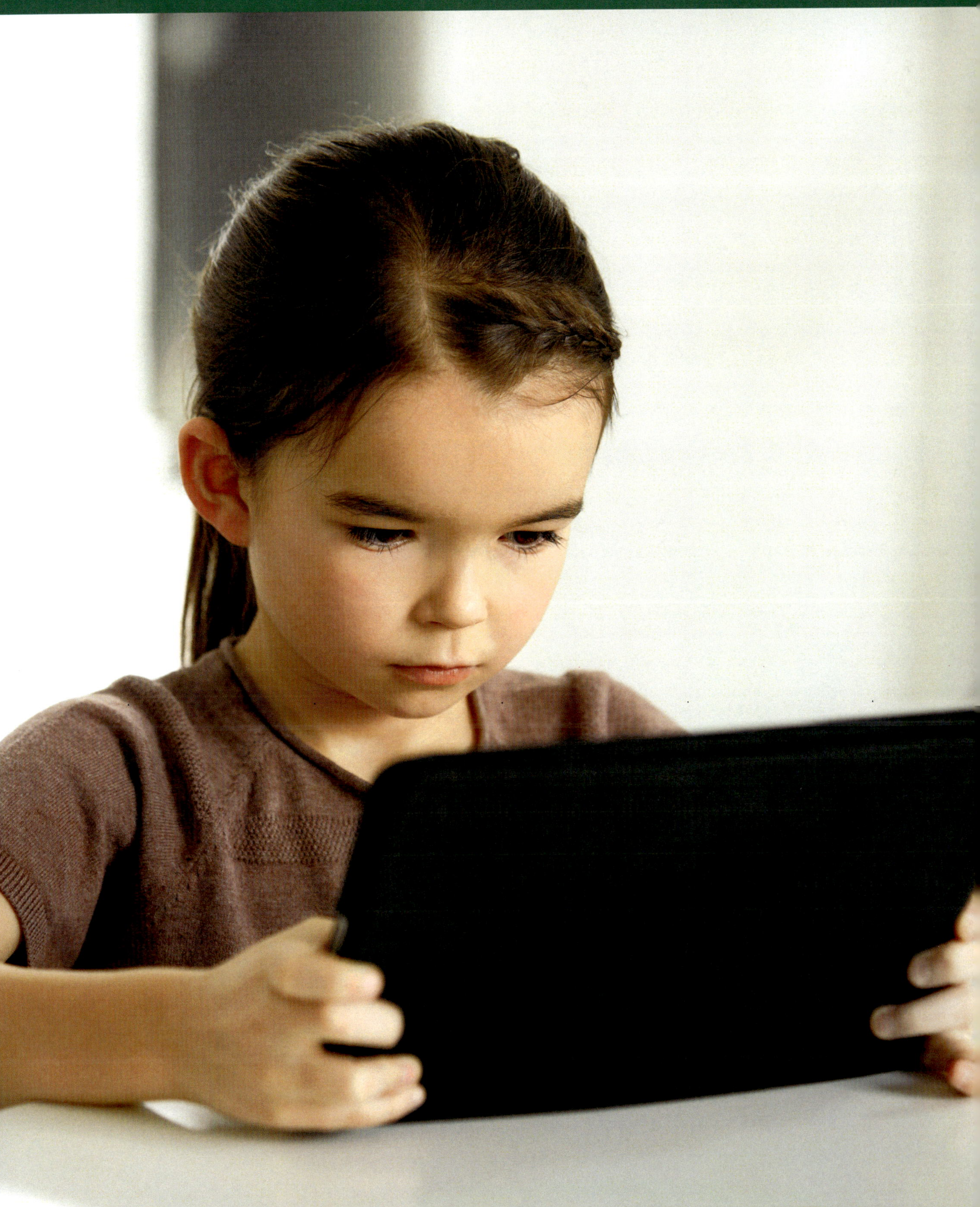

Digital Media
Part 2: Media Effects
Collection Introduction

Tiffany Munzer, MD, FAAP
Member of AAP Council on Communications and Media Executive Committee
Assistant Professor of Pediatrics; Division of Developmental Behavioral Pediatrics
University of Michigan, Ann Arbor, MI

Jenny Radesky, MD, FAAP
Chair, AAP Council on Communications and Media
Associate Professor of Pediatrics and Division Director, Developmental Behavioral Pediatrics
University of Michigan, Ann Arbor, MI

Part 2 of this series on digital media offers a natural transition from how systems are shaping children's digital media use, highlighting how digital media use might shape children's well-being. Pediatricians strive to shape and bend the arc of a child's development and health toward opportunity. As a specialty, pediatric providers are forward-thinking and anticipate the next developmental steps of their patients to provide the best evidence-based, anticipatory guidance. However, this task is at odds with the rapid pace of technological development and the amorphous unknowns of tomorrow. When we fast-forward decades into the future, the technological possibilities are so vast that they may be unpredictable to even the most prescient pediatrician.

As this introduction is being written, digital media companies are racing to leverage artificial intelligence (AI) technologies for commercial purposes. The evolution of technology continues without enough input from families and pediatricians to design the technology to suit children's needs. Indeed, as new technologies emerge, families embrace them at an increasingly faster rate.

However, previous media effects research can provide insights into the future. Part 2 of this book series reflects on earlier discoveries about the impact of digital media on child and adolescent outcomes. This collection includes research that illuminates the ways that digital media can introduce risks through harmful content, displacement of other healthy behaviors, or contact from unwanted adults. The scope of these papers includes how digital media intersects with physical health, such as sedentary behaviors and eating disorders. Additionally, this body of work has examined how digital media intersects with social determinants of health and mental health, such as online victimization, problematic internet use, and academic performance.

The focus of the works in Part 2 includes a problem-focused lens, an approach that traditional medical training has emphasized. However, this approach may miss the unique individual characteristics and the tailored, limitless affordances of digital media characteristics that are part of the nuance of families' online experiences. As precision medicine has revolutionized the study and treatment of individual conditions, a similarly personalized and tailored approach is being leveraged by digital media companies to keep young people engaged with their products and generate revenue.

As we look toward the future, developments in digital media technologies and AI will—and have already—create algorithms selecting commercialized content for children with surgical precision. We might expect a wider array of content that is even lower quality as a result of AI-generated content, with no thoughtful human at the helm to ensure content meets the developmental needs of children. We might expect sophisticated interactive designs to demand more timed play for young children. We might also expect AI to widen the systemic and structural disparities that unfortunately shape children's and adolescent's daily lives and digital experiences.

Screen Media Use and Academic Performance Among Children and Adolescents

Source: *Adelantado-Renau M, Moliner-Urdiales D, Cavero-Redondo I, et al. Association between screen media use and academic performance among children and adolescents: a systematic review and meta-analysis. JAMA Pediatr. 2019 23 September [published online ahead of print]; doi: 10.1001/jamapediatrics.2019.3176*

Investigators from institutions in multiple countries conducted a systematic review and meta-analysis to assess the association between academic performance and screen use (including television viewing, Internet surfing, video games, and mobile phone usage). The authors used a systematic methodology to identify relevant, published, cross-sectional studies that included children 4–18 years old; measured screen use by time or frequency; and assessed the association between screen use and academic performance as measured by grades, standardized tests, academic failure, or self-report on school performance. Data from studies included in the meta-analysis were used to assess the statistical association with academic performance. Outcomes for the statistical analyses included mathematics and language academic performance and a composite academic performance score. Analyses limited to children (4–11.9 years old) and adolescents (12–18 years old) were also conducted.

Data on 58 studies that included 480,479 participants were selected for the systematic review, and 30 of these studies, with a total of 106,653 participants, were included in the meta-analysis. Included studies were published between 1958 and 2018; 36 (62%) assessed the effects of television viewing, 23 (40%) video game playing, 9 (16%) Internet surfing, 5 (9%) mobile phone use, and 10 (17%) overall screen use. The results of studies included in the systematic review suggested a negative association between television viewing and academic performance, while results of studies on the association between video games and academic performance either suggested a negative association or no association with academic performance. Results of studies on Internet surfing were equivocal. There was no association found between mobile phone use and academic performance in the included studies.

In the meta-analysis, there was no statistical association between overall screen use and academic performance. However, increased television viewing was associated with statistically lower academic performance, including composite, language, and mathematics scores. There was also a statistical association between increased video game playing and lower composite scores. In subgroup analyses, television viewing was inversely and significantly associated with language and mathematics scores in children, and with mathematics and composite scores in adolescents. Increased video game playing was associated with significantly lower composite scores in adolescents.

The authors conclude that the effect of each type of screen use on academic performance should be assessed individually. Television viewing and video game playing appeared to be the activities with the most negative association with academic performance.

COMMENTARY BY

Benjamin R. Doolittle, MD, M Div, FAAP, FACP, Internal Medicine and Pediatrics, Yale School of Medicine, New Haven, CT

Dr Doolittle has disclosed no financial relationship relevant to this commentary. This commentary does not contain a discussion of an unapproved/investigative use of a commercial product/device.

Is all screen time equal? Based on the current investigation, the answer appears to be a qualified "no." Television viewing and video gaming were associated with lower academic scores, while smartphone use and total screen time were not. The proposed mechanism is the association of television viewing with reduced physical activity, verbal interaction, and mental effort.[1] Similarly, video gaming has been associated with emotional and behavioral health problems.[2]

We should be cautious about these findings. While smart phone use and total screen time were not associated with worse academic performance, several studies have shown negative correlations between total screen time and loneliness, depression, cardiovascular risks, sleep quality, and life satisfaction.[3–5] Investigators note the heterogeneity of results. For example, Internet use was associated with improved academic performance when used for educational purposes and poorer performance when used for entertainment. High Internet use and no Internet use were both associated with poorer performance.

The definition of "screen time" is complex. A child can passively watch a television program, video chat with friends, do homework, and play video games. Some activities may promote school performance, while others may detract. Even the nature of television viewing is changing. The earliest studies from 1949 demonstrated increased family cohesion: families watched television together.[6] Today, television serials are often watched on streaming services with personal devices. Confounding these questions is socioeconomic status. Children with more resources (computers, smart phones, etc) may perform better academically despite increased screen time. Further research will need to disentangle the nuanced quality and quantity of these screen time interactions.

Bottom Line: Increased television viewing and video gaming appear to be associated with lower academic performance. Total screen use and mobile phone use may not be associated with lower academic performance. The effect on performance of Internet surfing is equivocal.

EDITORS' NOTE

My mother realized in about 1957 that too much television was probably not good for children, frequently turning off our set and telling my siblings and me to "go play outside." I'm not sure that the science has progressed much since then. Although the meta-analysis in the current study demonstrated an association between television viewing and academic performance, association does not equal causation.

References available at https://doi.org/10.1542/gr.43-1-5.

Screening for Problematic Internet Use

Jonathan D'Angelo, PhD, Megan A. Moreno, MD, MSEd, MPH

abstract

Problematic Internet use (PIU) by adolescents is of growing concern among both parents and pediatricians. Early controversies may have contributed to challenges in defining and measuring PIU. A variety of screening tools have evolved, aligned with different constructs of PIU, although a validated screening tool does exist. Current data and American Academy of Pediatrics policy reflect evidence-driven screening for PIU for all youth.

University of Wisconsin–Madison, Madison, Wisconsin

Both authors approved the final manuscript as submitted and agree to be accountable for all aspects of the work.

DOI: https://doi.org/10.1542/peds.2019-2056F

Accepted for publication Jan 29, 2020

Address correspondence to Jonathan D'Angelo, PhD, Department of Pediatrics, University of Wisconsin–Madison, 2870 University Ave, Madison, WI 53705. E-mail: jddangelo@wisc.edu

PEDIATRICS (ISSN Numbers: Print, 0031-4005; Online, 1098-4275).

FINANCIAL DISCLOSURE: The authors have indicated they have no financial relationships relevant to this article to disclose.

FUNDING: No external funding.

POTENTIAL CONFLICT OF INTEREST: The authors have indicated they have no potential conflicts of interest to disclose.

ARTICLE

PROBLEMATIC INTERNET USE

Internet use is nearly ubiquitous among adolescents and young adults. Current US data suggest that 93% of adolescents and adults between 12 and 29 years of age go online, and up to 25% of teens describe themselves as "constantly connected."[1] Given these high rates of Internet use, problematic Internet use (PIU) is a growing concern.[2,3] Researchers have identified a rising number of consequences associated with increased Internet use among adolescents, including, but not limited to, psychological issues, behavior problems, attention problems, and physical problems.[4] Given that Internet use begins increasingly earlier in adolescence and even during the childhood years, pediatricians are uniquely positioned to conduct early screening for PIU.[5]

The Controversial History of PIU

An initial principle important to understanding this topic is the notion that Internet addiction and PIU represent different concepts. Although these terms have been used interchangeably in the past, they represent 2 separate frameworks for identifying Internet overuse. Internet addiction may be considered more analogous to a classic substance addiction, with loss of control and feelings of withdrawal. PIU represents a broader array of problems related to Internet use, including social, behavioral, and emotional issues.[6] An extreme case of PIU may involve Internet addiction, but PIU is a broader, more multifaceted concept.

Efforts toward developing diagnostic criteria for PIU began 2 decades ago. Reviewing the evolution of the concept of PIU illustrates the dilemma around whether PIU represents a behavioral addiction, impulsivity, or a broader range of behaviors. The focus on aspects of addictive behaviors likely stems from 2 initial approaches to defining PIU, grounded in existing *Diagnostic and Statistical Manual of Mental Disorders, Fourth Edition*, disorders: substance abuse and/or dependency and pathologic gambling.[7,8] After this early work came the introduction of 3 conceptual approaches. First, PIU was more broadly described as a general behavioral addiction.[9,10] Second, a cognitive-behavioral model of PIU drew attention to the impact of an individual's thoughts on his or her development of problematic behaviors and separated PIU into "generalized" PIU (or multidimensional overuse of the Internet) and "specific" PIU.[11] Specific PIU was defined as dependence on a specific function of the Internet, such as online shopping. Third, a model proposed that PIU should be more widely classified as an impulse control disorder with criteria, including maladaptive preoccupation with Internet use characterized by either irresistible use or use that is excessive and longer than planned, clinically significant distress or impairment, and the absence of other Axis I disorders.[12]

Current Definition of PIU

At present, the current definition of PIU arose from a previous study that was focused on developing stakeholder-driven consensus-based criteria. In this study, the authors used a concept mapping approach, which integrates qualitative and quantitative data from key stakeholders with expertise or investment in the topic. For this study, investigators incorporated data from researchers in the fields of adolescent health, addiction science, and technology, as well as from adolescents and young adults themselves. The authors identified 7 specific constructs within PIU: (1) psychosocial risk factors (ie, anxiety) that increase because of PIU behavior, (2) physical impairment, (3) emotional impairment, (4) social and/or functional impairment, (5) risky Internet use, (6) impulsive Internet use, and (7) dependent Internet use.[13] The strength of this definition is supported by its thorough review of the phenomenon as it may present among adolescents. From this study's findings, PIU was defined as "Internet use that is risky, excessive, or impulsive in nature, leading to adverse life consequences, specifically physical, emotional, social, or functional impairment."

It is important to note that PIU among adolescents goes beyond just spending too much time online. The definitions and constructs above represent both how much time is spent online (ie, the quantity of use) as well as the relationship with the online world, which represents quality of use.

It is estimated that 7% to 11% of adolescents in the United States suffer from PIU.[13-16] Hence, it is possible that it affects 1 in every 10 adolescent patients. This is a consequential statistic because PIU is associated with conduct problems (fighting), hyperactivity, symptoms of depression, a negative impact on daily functions and physical health,[17] trouble concentrating, suicidal ideation among women in college,[18] and poor interpersonal relationships.[19]

Screening for PIU

One of the more problematic aspects of PIU is the challenge of screening for it. In comparison to a dependence on a substance, PIU is a maladaptive relationship with tools that one needs to function in society. Hence, there are 3 strategies that can potentially serve to help identify patients with PIU: know the risk factors, use an established screening tool, and identify opportunities to screen.

Risk Factors for PIU

There are some categories of individuals who might be at higher risk for PIU. First, any of the associated consequences noted above may serve as indicators. This is because causal connections between PIU and Internet addiction and the various outcomes have yet to be strongly established in the literature.[20] Previous research supports that there are particular groups at increased risk, including males,[21–23] those who experience depressive symptoms and use the Internet for relationships and mood regulation,[24] adolescents with high levels of narcissism and the feeling of a need to belong,[25] and those who experience fear of missing out.[26] Family risk factors can also play a role, including adolescents who experience family dissatisfaction[22] and adolescents who have parents with mental health issues.[27]

Screening Tools for PIU

Given the number of different definitions proposed for PIU, it may not be surprising that a number of different tools have been developed to assess for PIU and Internet addiction.[17,28–30] However, a systematic review that was focused on PIU screening instruments illustrated that many tools were not supported by evidence. For example, most tools had one or more of the following flaws: they were designed for adults, used different conceptual foci than PIU, had varied or seemingly random cutoff points for indicating an at-risk individual, and had a lack of scientific validation for the tool.[31] One pediatric-focused validated screening tool for PIU is the Problematic and Risky Internet Use Screening Scale (PRIUSS),[15] an 18-item scale that has 3 distinct subscales: social impairment, emotional impairment, and risky and/or impulsive Internet use (see Supplemental Information). At present, this remains the only validated screening tool for pediatric populations.

Nonrecommended Screening Approaches for PIU

It is also important to point out a nonrecommended approach, which is to focus on time spent online. Whereas early screening approaches asked patients and families to report the number of hours of "screen time," the 2016 American Academy of Pediatrics (AAP) policy statement on media use in school-aged children and adolescents no longer recommends that strategy for this population.[32] This shift in screening focus represents newer evidence that illustrates time spent online is not the only factor involved in PIU as well as a lack of evidence to support strict hour-based recommendations that can apply across various developmental stages.

When To Screen for PIU

An opportune time to screen is during routine health supervision visits because many pediatricians use paper or digital screening tools to assess multiple behavioral concerns at these visits. The 18-item PRIUSS typically takes 5 minutes or less to complete; however, a shorter, validated screening tool is the 3-item PRIUSS, which has 3 questions regarding anxiety when away from the Internet, loss of motivation when on the Internet, and feelings of withdrawal when away from the Internet.[33] These 3 questions can be incorporated with other commonly used behavioral screening tools. Positive screens on the 3-item PRIUSS can be followed-up with the full scale, similar to the use of the Patient Health Questionnaire-2, which is commonly used to identify those who would benefit from screening with the Patient Health Questionnaire 9.

Other opportunities to screen children and adolescents may be in cases when parents are concerned about sleep patterns or have challenges in limiting screen time around bedtime. Children and adolescents who experience a dramatic change in grades may also benefit from screening.

The Role of the Pediatrician After Screening

Unfortunately, there are currently no evidence-based prevention strategies or interventions to rely on if a pediatric patient screens at risk for PIU. In absence of this evidence, one tool to consider is the Family Media Use Plan (https://www.healthychildren.org/english/media/pages/default.aspx), developed by the AAP. This tool allows families to view suggested structure and ideas for Internet and media use and select (or create) items that fit their families' needs and values. It also includes a "media time calculator" that allows individuals to consider a typical day's activities and how much media or Internet time fits in alongside critical health activities such as sleep and physical activities, social activities (ie, family or friend time), and academic activities (ie, school and homework). This tool can be used at any age, and it is recommended that the plan be reviewed and updated at least yearly or with changes in schedule (eg, school schedule to summer schedule). The Family Media Use Plan was developed alongside the 2016 AAP policy statement on media use among school-aged children and adolescents[32] in an effort to translate those evidence-based recommendations into a parent-facing tool.

Future Directions for Research

Given that PIU remains a newer pediatric concern, there are a number of important areas for future research. Much of the past research has been focused on developing different conceptual approaches and screening tools. More recently, there have been a number of new screening tools that are focused on different aspects of PIU. This includes screening tools specifically for social media addiction and smartphone addiction.[34,35] At this point, research has become semisaturated with new screening tools with little scientific validation or clinical usefulness. However, there is a dearth of research in the areas of prevention and intervention. Teenagers may tell pediatricians anecdotal reports of teachers who institute "screen-free weeks" or about their experiences with losing Internet access on summer vacation and how different they feel. These unpublished stories support the need for research to understand pediatric patients' experiences and leverage them for effective prevention and intervention approaches.

CONCLUSIONS

Although PIU is still a relatively new phenomenon, there is general agreement that it is a serious issue that adolescents face and can present patients with an array of negative consequences. It is important for pediatricians to understand this emerging literature, the risk factors, and how to screen and counsel to best support their patients.

> **ABBREVIATIONS**
>
> AAP: American Academy of Pediatrics
> PIU: problematic Internet use
> PRIUSS: Problematic and Risky Internet Screening Scale

REFERENCES

1. Lenhart APK, Smith A, Zickhur K. *Social Media and Young Adults*. Washington, DC: Pew Internet and American Life Project; 2010
2. Christakis DA, Moreno MA. Trapped in the net: will internet addiction become a 21st-century epidemic? *Arch Pediatr Adolesc Med*. 2009;163(10):959–960
3. Dell'Osso B, Altamura AC, Allen A, Marazziti D, Hollander E. Epidemiologic and clinical updates on impulse control disorders: a critical review. *Eur Arch Psychiatry Clin Neurosci*. 2006;256(8):464–475
4. Rosen LD, Lim AF, Felt J, et al. Media and technology use predicts ill-being among children, preteens and teenagers independent of the negative health impacts of exercise and eating habits. *Comput Human Behav*. 2014;35:364–375
5. Jelenchick LA, Christakis DA. Problematic internet use during adolescence and young adulthood. In: Strasburger VC, Moreno MA, eds. *AM: STARs Social Networking & New Technologies: Adolescent Medicine State of the Art Review*. Itasca, IL: American Academy of Pediatrics; 2014:605–620
6. Cheever NA, Moreno MA, Rosen LD. When does internet and smartphone use become a problem? In: Moreno MA, Radovic A, eds. *Technology and Adolescent Mental Health*. New York, NY: Springer; 2018:121–131
7. Young KS. Psychology of computer use: XL. Addictive use of the Internet: a case that breaks the stereotype. *Psychol Rep*. 1996;79(3 pt 1):899–902
8. Young KS. Internet addiction: the emergence of a new clinical disorder. *Cyberpsychol Behav*. 1998;1(3):237–244
9. Griffiths M. Internet addiction: fact or fiction? *Psychologist*. 1999;12(5):246–250
10. Grant JE, Potenza MN, Weinstein A, Gorelick DA. Introduction to behavioral addictions. *Am J Drug Alcohol Abuse*. 2010;36(5):233–241
11. Davis RA. A cognitive-behavioral model of pathological Internet use. *Comput Human Behav*. 2001;17(2):187–195
12. Shapira NA, Lessig MC, Goldsmith TD, et al. Problematic internet use: proposed classification and diagnostic criteria. *Depress Anxiety*. 2003;17(4):207–216
13. Moreno MA, Jelenchick LA, Christakis DA. Problematic internet use among older adolescents: a conceptual framework. *Comput Human Behav*. 2013;29(4):1879–1887
14. Jelenchick LA, Hawk ST, Moreno MA. Problematic Internet use and social networking site use among Dutch adolescents. *Int J Adolesc Med Health*. 2016;28(1):119–121
15. Jelenchick LA, Eickhoff J, Christakis DA, et al. The Problematic and Risky Internet Use Screening Scale (PRIUSS) for adolescents and young adults: scale development and refinement. *Comput Human Behav*. 2014;35:171–178
16. Jelenchick LA, Christakis DA, Moreno MA. A longitudinal evaluation of problematic Internet use (PIU) symptoms in older adolescents. In: Proceedings from the 2014 Pediatric Academic Society; May 3–7, 2014; Vancouver, British Columbia, Canada
17. Aboujaoude E. Problematic Internet use: an overview. *World Psychiatry*. 2010;9(2):85–90
18. Moreno MA, Jelenchick LA, Breland DJ. Exploring depression and problematic internet use among college females: a multisite study. *Comput Human Behav*. 2015;49:601–607
19. Milani L, Osualdella D, Di Blasio P. Quality of interpersonal relationships and problematic Internet use in adolescence. *Cyberpsychol Behav*. 2009;12(6):681–684
20. Cerniglia L, Zoratto F, Cimino S, Laviola G, Ammaniti M, Adriani W. Internet addiction in adolescence: neurobiological, psychosocial and clinical issues. *Neurosci Biobehav Rev*. 2017;76(pt A):174–184
21. Stavropoulos V, Alexandraki K, Motti-Stefanidi F. Recognizing internet addiction: prevalence and relationship to academic achievement in adolescents enrolled in urban and rural Greek high schools. *J Adolesc*. 2013;36(3):565–576
22. Lam LT, Peng Z-W, Mai J-C, Jing J. Factors associated with Internet addiction among adolescents. *Cyberpsychol Behav*. 2009;12(5):551–555
23. Widyanto L, Griffiths M. 'Internet addiction': a critical review. *Int J Ment Health Addict*. 2006;4(1):31–51
24. Gámez-Guadix M. Depressive symptoms and problematic Internet use among adolescents: analysis of the longitudinal relationships from the cognitive-behavioral model. *Cyberpsychol Behav Soc Netw*. 2014;17(11):714–719
25. Casale S, Fioravanti G. Why narcissists are at risk for developing Facebook addiction: the need to be admired and the need to belong. *Addict Behav*. 2018;76:312–318

26. Oberst U, Wegmann E, Stodt B, Brand M, Chamarro A. Negative consequences from heavy social networking in adolescents: the mediating role of fear of missing out. *J Adolesc.* 2017;55: 51–60

27. Lam LT. Parental mental health and Internet addiction in adolescents. *Addict Behav.* 2015;42:20–23

28. Chen SH, Weng LJ, Su YJ, Wu HM, Yang PF. Development of a Chinese Internet addiction scale and its psychometric study. *Chin J Psychol.* 2003;45(3): 279–294

29. Ko C-H, Yen J-Y, Yen C-F, Chen C-C, Yen C-N, Chen S-H. Screening for Internet addiction: an empirical study on cut-off points for the Chen Internet Addiction Scale. *Kaohsiung J Med Sci.* 2005; 21(12):545–551

30. Young KS. *Caught in the Net: How to Recognize the Signs of Internet Addiction–and a Winning Strategy for Recovery.* New York, NY: John Wiley & Sons; 1998

31. Kuss DJ, Griffiths MD, Karila L, Billieux J. Internet addiction: a systematic review of epidemiological research for the last decade. *Curr Pharm Des.* 2014;20(25): 4026–4052

32. Council on Communications and Media. Media use in school-aged children and adolescents. *Pediatrics.* 2016;138(5): e20162592

33. Moreno MA, Arseniev-Koehler A, Selkie E. Development and testing of a 3-item screening tool for problematic Internet use. *J Pediatr.* 2016;176: 167–172.e1

34. Csibi S, Demetrovics Z, Szabó A. [Development and psychometric validation of the Brief Smartphone Addiction Scale (BSAS) with schoolchidren]. *Psychiatr Hung.* 2016; 31(1):71–77

35. Bányai F, Zsila Á, Király O, et al. Problematic social media use: results from a large-scale nationally representative adolescent sample. *PLoS One.* 2017;12(1): e0169839

Cyberbullying and Eating Disorders

Source: *Cheng CM, Chu J, Ganson KT, et al. Cyberbullying and eating disorder symptoms in US early adolescents. Published online ahead of print September 6, 2023. Int J Eat Disord; doi:10.1002/eat.24034.*

Investigators from multiple institutions conducted an analysis to assess the relationship between cyberbullying, either as a victim or perpetrator, and eating disorder symptoms in early adolescents. For the study, they analyzed data from the year 2 follow-up of the Adolescent Brain Cognitive Development (ABCD) study. ABCD is a longitudinal study assessing brain development and health in 11,875 youths recruited from 21 sites across the US. Participants in the current analysis were youths 10–14 years old with data on cyberbullying and eating disorder symptoms. Cyberbullying victimization or perpetration was determined by self-report to 2 items in the 2-year follow-up ABCD questionnaire. Eating disorder symptoms were classified using the Kiddie Schedule for Affective Disorders and Schizophrenia (KSADS-5), a computerized tool for categorizing mental health concerns based on Diagnostic and Statistical Manual, 5th Edition (DSM-5) criteria. Using KSADS-5 responses, participants were classified as having specific eating disorder symptoms, including worry about weight gain, self-worth tied to weight, inappropriate compensatory behaviors to lose weight (only eating foods with minimal calories, exercising a lot, throwing up, and taking diuretics, laxatives, or diet pills), binge eating, and distress with binge eating. Separate Poisson regression models were used to assess the relationship between either cyberbullying victimization or perpetration and each of the specific eating disorder symptoms. Demographic characteristics such as sex, race/ethnicity, household income, and parental education level were included in the regression models, and responses were weighted to provide nationally representative results.

Data were analyzed on 10,258 youths, with a mean age of 12.0 ±0.1 years. The prevalence of self-reported cyberbullying victimization and perpetration was 9.5% and 1.1%, respectively. Rates of eating disorder symptoms were 1.45% for worry about weight gain, 1.67% for self-worth tied to weight, 6.51% for inappropriate compensatory behaviors to lose weight, 7.50% for binge eating, and 2.89% for distress with binge eating. Compared to those who did not report being cyberbullied, cyberbullying victimization was significantly associated with worry about weight gain (prevalence ratio [PR], 2.41; 95% confidence interval [CI], 1.48, 3.91), inappropriate compensatory behaviors to lose weight (PR, 1.95; 95% CI, 1.57, 2.42), binge eating (PR, 1.95; 95% CI, 1.59, 2.39), and distress about binge eating (PR, 2.64; 95% CI, 1.94, 3.59). Cyberbullying perpetration was associated with a significantly increased risk for worry about weight gain (PR, 3.52; 95% CI, 1.19, 3.07), self-worth tied to weight (PR, 5.59; 95% CI, 2.56, 12.20), binge eating (PR, 2.36; 95% CI, 1.44, 3.87), and distress with binge eating (PR, 2.84; 95% CI, 1.47, 5.49).

The authors conclude that self-reported cyberbullying victimization and perpetration in early adolescence were associated with eating disorder symptoms.

COMMENTARY BY

Meghna Raphael, MD, FAAP, Adolescent Medicine and Sports Medicine, Texas Children's Hospital, Baylor College of Medicine, Houston, TX

Dr Raphael has disclosed no financial relationship relevant to this commentary. This commentary does not contain a discussion of an unapproved/investigative use of a commercial product/device.

Cyberbullying is pervasive and occurs even in spaces that adolescents may have thought to be safe.[1] In a 2021 national survey of more than 1,300 youths, 42% of 10-year-olds, 71% of 12-year-olds, and 91% of 14-year-olds owned a personal smartphone.[2] When considering tablets and computers, device access and hence possible exposure to cyberbullying among adolescents is widespread.[2]

Potential confounders that were not reported in the current cross-sectional study include: possible differences in smartphone ownership, the manner of device use, differences in screentime, and extent of social media use among the 2 groups studied. While social media use is increasing, it is not universal. Nearly 62% of 8–12-year-olds and 16% of 13–18-year-olds report never using social media.[2] Conceivably, adolescents in the current study who were victims or perpetrators of cyberbullying were using their devices to communicate or were using social media. Besides cyberbullying, adolescents with greater social media use may also be exposed to other factors that can influence the development of eating disorder symptoms. These include frequent exposure to an "idealized body image" from peers or influencers and increased access to inaccurate information about nutrition or exercise regimens. In the case of highly visual platforms (eg, Instagram or Snapchat), the use of filters and editing tools while posting pictures also can lead to body dissatisfaction.[2] Hence, if social media use was higher in adolescents exposed to cyberbullying, this may have been independently related to eating disorder symptoms. Additionally, reporting bias needs to be considered in the current study. It is possible that adolescents would be unlikely to admit to cyberbullying perpetration even in an anonymous survey.

Despite these limitations, the current study investigators reinforce existing knowledge on the potential adverse effects of cyberbullying victimization and perpetration on the emergence of eating disorder symptoms. As eating disorder symptoms can be present for several months prior to recognition of the disease, and symptoms of anorexia nervosa often begin in early adolescence (See *AAP Grand Rounds*. 2022;48[6]:65),[4] an important strength of the current study is the inclusion of younger adolescents.

Bottom Line: Cyberbullying in young adolescents necessitates screening for eating disorder symptoms.

References

1. Selkie EM, et al. *J Adolesc Health*. 2016;58(2):125-133; doi: 10.1016/j.jadohealth.2015.09.026.
2. Rideout V, et al. Common Sense census: Media use by tweens and teens, 2021. San Francisco, CA: Common Sense.https://www.commonsensemedia.org/research/the-common-sense-census-media-use-by-tweens-and-teens-2021. March 9, 2022.
3. Sharma A, Vidal C. *J Eat Disord*. 2023;11(1):170; doi: 10.1186/s40337-023-00898-6.
4. Ranzenhofer LM, et al. *J Adolesc Health*. 2022;71(5):587-593; doi: 10.1016/j.jadohealth.2022.06.010.

in Brief

What Pediatricians Should Know and Do about Cyberbullying

Jane Timmons-Mitchell, PhD,* Daniel J. Flannery, PhD*
*Begun Center for Violence Prevention, Research and Education, Jack, Joseph and Morton Mandel School of Applied Social Sciences, Case Western Reserve University, Cleveland, OH

AUTHOR DISCLOSURE Drs Timmons-Mitchell and Flannery have disclosed no financial relationships relevant to this article. This commentary does not contain a discussion of an unapproved/investigative use of a commercial product/device.

The Impact of Social Media on Children, Adolescents, and Families. Schurgin O'Keeffe G, Clarke-Pearson K; Council on Communications and Media. *Pediatrics.* 2011;127(4):800–804

A Comprehensive Technical Package for the Prevention of Youth Violence and Associated Risk Behaviors. David-Ferdon C, Vivolo-Kantor AM, Dahlberg LL, et al. Atlanta, GA: National Center for Injury Prevention and Control, Centers for Disease Control and Prevention; 2016.

Bullying Prevention: A Summary of the Report of the National Academies of Sciences, Engineering, and Medicine. Flannery DJ, Todres J, Bradshaw CP, et al. *Prev Sci.* 2016;17(8):1044–1053

Ask Suicide-Screening Questions (ASQ): A Brief Instrument for the Pediatric Emergency Department. Horowitz, LM, Bridge, JA, Teach, SJ, et al. *Arch Pediatr Adolesc Med.* 2012;166(12):1170–1176

StopBullying.gov website. US Department of Health and Human Services. http://www.stopbullying.gov. Accessed May 27, 2019

When bullying occurs through technology it is called *electronic bullying* or *cyberbullying*, which first appeared at the beginning of the 21st century and has become an issue of great concern to pediatricians, parents, educators, and youths themselves. Although cyberbullying includes aspects of traditional, in-person bullying, it also differs in important respects. The Centers for Disease Control and Prevention (CDC) defines bullying as any unwanted aggressive behavior(s) by another youth or group of youths who are not siblings or current dating partners that involves an observed or perceived power imbalance and is repeated multiple times or is highly likely to be repeated. Bullying, whether in-person or through technology, can inflict distress on the targeted youth, as well as physical, psychological, social, or educational harm.

Cyberbullying should be considered in the context of traditional bullying rather than as a separate entity: it shares characteristics with traditional forms of bullying, such as its risk factors, its negative consequences, and the effectiveness of interventions that work on both types bullying. But there are also important differences between the 2: cyberbullying does not always have a clearly defined power differential, and 1 negative post can have significant effects without being repeated by its perpetrator.

Estimates of the frequency of cyberbullying vary. The CDC indicates that more than 15% of high school students report being cyberbullied in the past year. Other estimates include a range from 4% to 90%, with many studies reporting 20% to 40%. Rates of cyberbullying perpetration range from 3% to 36%. In 1 study, when parents were asked about their child's cyberbullying experiences, 80% of parents claimed that they were knowledgeable about their child's online behavior, but 89% did not know that their child had reported being cyberbullied. Many youths (approximately one-third) who are cyberbullied have also been victims of traditional bullying. Of concern is the estimate that only approximately half of youth who are cyberbullied seek help by reporting the occurrence to anyone.

Although some studies report that girls are more likely than boys to be targets of cyberbullying, others suggest that boys and girls are targeted at equal rates. Sexual and gender minority youths are targeted more frequently than their peers, as are racial and ethnic minority youths.

Well-designed studies have identified many harmful effects of cyberbullying. Being a victim of cyberbullying has been shown to increase the likelihood of psychological distress, including depression. Compared with nonvictims, youths who were victims of cyberbullying and/or traditional bullying reported 4 times the depressive symptoms and 5 times greater likelihood to make a suicide attempt. Unfortunately, one of the frequent causes of cyberbullying, relationship problems or a breakup, is further exacerbated by the bullying: youths who are victims of cyberbullying report increased social isolation and difficulty trusting others, especially peers.

One of the things that may distinguish cyberbullies from those who bully in-person is the belief that they can post anonymously with impunity, that offensive material cannot be traced back to them. What they might not realize is that they are creating digital footprints each time they go online. Although some forms of social media are more difficult to trace than others, cyber posts are not, in fact, anonymous. The Library of Congress, for example, is archiving everything posted on Twitter. Increasingly, Transportation Safety Administration agents seize cell phones at ports of entry. Sharing the reality that online behavior is not reliably anonymous is potentially a means to discourage inappropriate posts: the possibility of being identified as the author of a hurtful bullying message may provide an incentive to inhibit such posts.

In 2011, the American Academy of Pediatrics (AAP) released a clinical report on "The Impact of Social Media on Children, Adolescents, and Families." The report reviewed the benefits as well as the risks of social media use, concluding that cyberbullying is one of the biggest risks. The AAP recommends 4 courses of action for pediatricians: 1) advise parents to talk with their children about online use; 2) advise parents to learn about technology use so that they are comfortable and knowledgeable about social media when talking with their children; 3) discuss the creation of a family online use plan and institute family meetings to review it; and 4) advise parents to supervise their children's online activities actively and personally rather than just relying on computer-based programs to monitor.

At office visits, pediatricians should attend to the warning signs that a child is the victim of cyberbullying: increased somatic complaints, social withdrawal, school absenteeism, declining grades, behavioral outbursts, and suicidal ideation. If there is concern about the child's safety, a concern the child is in imminent danger, has been or might become the victim of physical or sexual abuse, or a concern about suicide, the pediatrician must contact the appropriate law enforcement authorities, the school, or an appropriate mental health professional; the child may need to be transported to the emergency department. Of course, screening for all of these issues is time-consuming and beyond the scope of many pediatric health supervision visits. Tools such as the HEEADDSSS (Home, Education, Eating, Activities, Drugs and Alcohol, Suicide and Depression, Sexuality and Safety) may be useful; the important thing is for the pediatrician to gather more information about the context and importance of possible symptoms. A brief screening instrument, the Ask Suicide-Screening Questions, has recently been developed and validated by the National Institute of Mental Health. The instrument, available without charge, takes less than 2 minutes to administer. If a youth screens positively, the Brief Suicide Safety Assessment can be administered by a physician or an assistant trained to use the protocol. A range of interventions, if needed, can be initiated in the pediatric office; referrals to other providers, such as psychologists or social workers, may be needed to continue in-depth assessment and to address the effects of cyberbullying.

If the child is a victim of cyberbullying, the pediatrician can recommend the following:

1. Don't forward, respond to, or "like" content that is harmful to others.
2. Keep evidence of cyberbullying, such as dates, times, descriptions, screen shots, e-mails, and texts.
3. Block the cyberbully.
4. Talk to a trusted adult.
5. Report bullying to the school and law enforcement as appropriate.

At a more general level, the pediatrician should incorporate how to be a good digital citizen into age-appropriate education. Parents should be encouraged to be aware of what their children are doing online and to talk with their children about how text and other online content can be perceived and the very real-world consequences of it. Parents need to remind children that digital content can spread quickly and explain what to do if they or someone else is being victimized by a cyberbully.

Most young people have access to digital media beginning in elementary school, and the trend is likely to increase. Although this access can be an important social and educational tool, it can also expose children to cyberbullying. Active parental supervision is needed, which can be reinforced by the pediatrician.

COMMENTS: Not infrequently, my wife and I, sitting in a restaurant, have noticed a couple (usually younger than we are) deeply engaged in their separate smartphones, making no eye contact with each other. Social media are overtaking social intimacy. Like drone warfare distancing the attacker from the attacked, cyberbullying is made easier by isolating the bully from the victim—no risk of eye contact. Once children played board games, sitting across from each other at a table; now the more usual is to interact through a screen—a word that is ironically apt. Time spent with video games is replacing outdoor activity, and well-developed thumbs are becoming more common than well-exercised bodies. Technology is radically changing the ways we relate (or don't) to each other; and, as yet, we are only slowly learning the implications. Akin to the invention of the printing press or the steam engine, we are moving into a (brave?) new world: *"And what rough beast, its hour come round at last, Slouches toward Bethlehem to be born?" (W.B. Yeats)*

—Henry M. Adam, MD
Associate Editor, *In Brief*

PS: On July 29, 2019, the front page of the *New York Times* Sports Section featured an article about Arthur Ashe Tennis Stadium being taken over the past weekend by thousands of fans paying to watch on huge screens 100 competitors vying for a $3 million first prize at the video game Fortnite. Brave new world indeed!

24-Hour Movement Behaviors and Impulsivity

Michelle D. Guerrero, PhD,[a] Joel D. Barnes, MSc,[a] Jeremy J. Walsh, PhD,[a,b] Jean-Philippe Chaput, PhD,[a,c,d] Mark S. Tremblay, PhD,[a,c] Gary S. Goldfield, PhD[a,c,d,e]

abstract

BACKGROUND: The objective of this study was to examine individual and concurrent associations between meeting the Canadian 24-Hour Movement Guidelines for Children and Youth (9–11 hours of sleep per night, ≤2 hours of recreational screen time (ST) per day, and at least 60 minutes of moderate to vigorous physical activity per day) and dimensions of impulsivity.

METHODS: Data from this cross-sectional observational study were part of the first annual curated release of the Adolescent Brain Cognitive Development Study. Participants included 4524 children between the ages of 8 and 11 years.

RESULTS: In analyses, it was shown that adherence to individual movement behavior recommendations as well as combinations of adherence to movement behavior recommendations were associated with each dimension of impulsivity. Meeting all 3 movement behavior recommendations was associated with lower positive urgency (95% confidence interval [CI]: −0.12 to −0.05), negative urgency (95% CI: −0.04 to −0.08), Behavioral Inhibition System (95% CI: −0.08 to −0.01), greater perseverance (95% CI: 0.09 to 0.15), and better scores on delay-discounting (95% CI: 0.57 to 0.94). Meeting the ST and sleep recommendations was associated with less impulsive behaviors on all dimensions of impulsivity: negative urgency (95% CI: −0.20 to −0.10), positive urgency (95% CI: −0.16 to −0.08), perseverance (95% CI: 0.06 to 0.15), Behavioral Inhibition System (95% CI: −0.15 to −0.03), Behavioral Activation System (BAS) reward responsiveness (95% CI: −0.04 to −0.05), BAS drive (95% CI: −0.14 to −0.06), BAS fun-seeking (95% CI: −0.15 to −0.17), and delay-discounting task (95% CI: 0.68 to 0.97).

CONCLUSIONS: Findings support efforts to determine if limiting recreational ST while promoting adequate sleep enhances the treatment and prevention of impulsivity-related disorders.

[a]Healthy Active Living and Obesity Research Group, Children's Hospital of Eastern Ontario Research Institute, Ottawa, Ontario, Canada; [b]Exercise, Metabolism, and Inflammation Laboratory, University of British Columbia Okanagan, Kelowna, British Columbia, Canada; and [c]Department of Pediatrics and [d]School of Human Kinetics, Faculty of Health Sciences, and [e]School of Psychology, Faculty of Social Sciences, University of Ottawa, Ottawa, Ontario, Canada

Dr Guerrero conceived the analytical approach, conducted all analyses, and assisted with drafting the initial manuscript; Mr Barnes and Drs Walsh, Chaput, and Tremblay assisted with data analysis and interpretation and critically reviewed the manuscript for important intellectual content; Dr Goldfield conceptualized the study, assisted with drafting the initial manuscript, and critically reviewed the manuscript for important intellectual content; and all authors approved the final manuscript as submitted and agree to be accountable for all aspects of the work.

DOI: https://doi.org/10.1542/peds.2019-0187

Accepted for publication Jun 10, 2019

Address correspondence to Dr Michelle D. Guerrero, PhD, Healthy Active Living and Obesity Research Group, Children's Hospital of Eastern Ontario Research Institute, 401 Smyth Rd, Ottawa, ON K1H 8L1, Canada. E-mail: mguerrero@cheo.on.ca

WHAT'S KNOWN ON THIS SUBJECT: Impulsivity has been implicated in the development and maintenance of psychiatric conditions. Sleep, screen time (ST), and physical activity have been independently associated with impulsivity among children; however, how these modifiable factors concurrently relate to children's impulse control is unknown.

WHAT THIS STUDY ADDS: This study is the first to show that adequate sleep and reduced ST are linked with less impulsive behavior among children. Efforts to determine if promoting adequate sleep and limiting ST enhances the prevention of impulsivity-related disorders are needed.

To cite: Guerrero MD, Barnes JD, Walsh JJ, et al. 24-Hour Movement Behaviors and Impulsivity. *Pediatrics.* 2019; 144(3):e20190187

ARTICLE

Impulsivity is often characterized as a tendency to act without forethought or to make decisions that reflect an inability to delay gratification; it is a multidimensional construct that encompasses cognitive, emotional, personality, and behavioral elements.[1] Impulsivity is a core characteristic in attention-deficit/hyperactivity disorder[2] but has also been implicated in the development and maintenance of many other psychiatric conditions, such as substance abuse disorders,[3,4] behavioral addictions,[5] eating disorders,[6] and other externalizing behavioral disorders.[7,8] Impulsivity has also been linked to emotion dysregulation leading to self-harm[9] and suicidal attempts among youth.[10] Thus, identifying modifiable determinants of impulsivity can inform targets to enhance the treatment and prevention of impulse control–related psychiatric disorders.

The average amount of sleep (in hours) that youth are achieving per night has decreased in recent decades, in part because of increased use of electronics.[11] Lack of sleep is related to greater impulsivity,[12] with mechanistic evidence suggesting that poor sleep negatively affects prefrontal cortical functioning, resulting in impairments in behavioral inhibition.[13] However, little data exist on the relationship between sleep duration and measures of impulsive personality traits and behavioral inhibition in preadolescent children.

It has been postulated that engaging with electronic devices during development (eg, smartphones), which often necessitates immediate responding to maintain communication or gaming, stimulates powerful behavioral and neurobiological (ie, dopamine release) reinforcement that promotes greater use, resulting in impaired inhibitory control, perseverance, emotion regulation, and other self-regulatory cognitive processes.[14] General support of these hypotheses has been found in several studies; weak impulse control has been associated with heavy engagement with mobile devices,[15] heavy media multitasking,[16] and excessive television watching (>3 hours per day).[13] However, most of this research has been conducted with older adolescents, and therefore relations among screen use and impulsivity in prepubertal children (8–11 years) are unclear.

Physical activity (PA) has been shown to improve domains of cognition,[17] including sustained attention, emotion regulation, and working memory, which are intricately associated with impulse control.[18] Thus, PA may be a viable method for promoting better inhibitory control and reducing impulsivity. Low levels of PA have been linked to impulsive behavior,[13] and it has been shown in several experimental studies that PA reduces behavioral inhibition among youth from clinical populations.[19,20] However, associations with other measures of impulsivity, such as delay-discounting (choosing smaller immediate rewards over larger more-delayed rewards) or self-reported impulsivity traits, have not been well studied in community samples of preadolescent children.

The Canadian 24-Hour Movement Guidelines for Children and Youth[21] are the first evidence-based movement guidelines that address an entire day. These guidelines recommend that children ages 5 to 13 years accumulate a minimum of 60 minutes per day in moderate to vigorous PA, spend no more than 2 hours per day in recreational screen time (ST), and obtain 9 to 11 hours of sleep per night. Children who meet all 3 movement behavior recommendations have better cognitive function,[22] lower odds of obesity,[23] better dietary patterns,[24] and enhanced quality of life[25] than children who do not meet any of the recommendations. Although individual 24-hour movement behaviors are important to consider in relation to impulsivity, what remains unknown is how these behaviors may concurrently relate to impulsivity in children. Therefore, the purpose of the current study was to examine if meeting the 24-hour movement behaviors individually and/or concurrently relate to a broad scope of dimensions of impulsivity in a large and diverse community sample of US children. We hypothesized that children who meet the movement behavior recommendations would exhibit lower scores on multiple indicators of impulsivity than those who do not meet recommendations and that meeting all recommendations would have the strongest relationship with impulsivity dimensions.

METHODS

Study Population

Participants were part of the Adolescent Brain Cognitive Development (ABCD) Study, an ongoing longitudinal, observational study on children's brain development and health.[26] Data for this study are collected on a biennial to annual basis over a 10-year period across 21 sites throughout the United States, using probabilistic sampling to obtain a large, diverse, and geographically stratified population-based sample. We used the first (baseline) cross-sectional curated release of the ABCD Study data set, which comprised 4524 children aged 8 to 11 years. Approval from all relevant institutional research ethics boards were obtained, along with signed informed consent from parents or guardians and assent from participating children in accordance with the principles of Helsinki. Information on the sample, recruitment, measure selection, and compensation are outlined elsewhere.[27,28]

Exposures

Sleep, ST, and PA served as the independent variables. Sleep was assessed by using one question from the Parent Sleep Disturbance Scale for Children.[29] Parents were asked to record the number of hours of sleep their child accumulated most nights. Recreational ST was measured by using the Youth Screen Time Survey (12 items),[30] wherein children were asked to report the number of hours spent engaged in screen-based activities (eg, watching shows and movies, texting) on a typical weekday and weekend day. Daily recreational ST was calculated by taking a weighted average of the weekday and weekend ST items: (sum of weekday ST in decimal hours × 5) + (sum of weekend day ST in decimal hours × 2)/7. PA was assessed by using one item from the Youth Risk Behavior Survey,[31] wherein children were asked to indicate on how many days they were active for at least 60 minutes per day in the last 7 days. Single-item measures of sleep and PA have moderate to strong criterion validity with accelerometry-assessed sleep and PA.[32,33]

Outcomes

Dimensions of impulsivity served as the outcome variables and were measured by using 3 child-reported assessments: UPPS-P Impulsive Behavior Scale[34] (D. Lynam, PhD, unpublished observations), Behavioral Inhibition System (BIS)/ Behavioral Activation System (BAS) Scale,[35] and cash choice delay-discounting task.[36] The UPPS-P scale comprises 5 dimensions: negative urgency (eg, "When I am upset, I often act without thinking"), positive urgency (eg, "When I get really happy about something, I tend to do things that can lead to trouble"), (lack of) premeditation (eg, "I like to stop and think things over before I do them"), (lack of) perseverance ("I finish what I start"), and sensation seeking (eg, "I like new, thrilling things, even if they are a little scary"). All items were scored on a 4-point Likert scale, anchored at 1 (not at all like me) and 4 (very much like me). Items assessing (lack of) premeditation and one item assessing (lack of) perseverance were reverse coded. High scores on negative and positive urgency indicate high impulsivity, whereas a high score on perseverance indicates low impulsivity. The BIS/ BAS Scale comprises 4 dimensions assessing BIS (eg, "I feel worried when I have done poorly at something"), BAS drive (eg, "I do everything to get the things that I want"), BAS reward responsiveness (eg, "I feel excited and full of energy when I get something that I want"), and BAS fun-seeking (eg, "I crave excitement and new sensations"). Items are scored on a 4-point Likert scale anchored at 0 (not true) and 3 (very true). For the delay-discounting task, children were asked to respond to a hypothetical question, indicating whether they would rather obtain $75 in 3 days (smaller, sooner reward) or $115 in 3 months (larger, later reward). They were also given a third "can't decide" option. Scores on the UPPS-P and BIS/BAS scales have been shown to have adequate reliability coefficients,[27] and the delay-discounting task has correlated well with real monetary rewards.[37]

Statistical Analyses

All analyses were conducted by using Mplus 8.2.[38] Missing data (<1%) were replaced by using multiple imputation. Robust full-information maximum likelihood estimation was used to account for possible nonnormality in responses. Confirmatory factor analyses (measurement models) were first conducted to examine the factorial structure of the UPPS-P and BIS/BAS scales. Intraclass correlations were calculated to determine if meaningful between-level (ie, data collection sites) differences affected the within-

TABLE 1 Means, SDs, and Composite Reliabilities of Study Variables

Variable	Mean	SD	CR
UPPS-P and BIS/BAS dimensions			
Negative urgency	2.10	0.65	0.63
Positive urgency	1.96	0.73	0.68
Perseverance	3.27	0.54	0.70
BIS	2.21	0.60	0.63
BAS drive	2.04	0.76	0.78
BAS reward responsiveness	3.22	0.57	0.74
BAS fun-seeking	2.44	0.65	0.65
Descriptives			
Age, y	10.00	0.61	NA
BMI, kg/m^2	18.63	3.94	NA
Family income[a]	7.41	2.28	NA
Parental education[b]	4.74	1.59	NA

CR, composite reliability; NA, not applicable.

[a] Combined income in past 12 mo from all sources before taxes and deductions on a scale of 1 to 10. 1 = ≤ $5000; 2 = $5000–$11 199; 3 = $12 000–$15 999; 4 = $16 000–$24 999; 5 = $25 000–$34 999; 6 = $35 000–$49 999; 7 = $50 000–$74 999; 8 = $75 000–$99 999; 9 = $100 000–$199 999; and 10 = ≥$200 000 (all in US dollars).

[b] Highest score on a scale of 1 to 7. 1 = ≤ grade 12; 2 = high school graduate or General Educational Development certification; 3 = some college; 4 = associate degree; 5 = bachelor's degree; 6 = master's degree; and 7 = professional or doctorate degree.

level dependent variables. The intraclass correlations from the unconditional models were low (ranged from 0.003 to 0.03), suggesting that there was little variability between data collection sites. Therefore, although the data were treated as nonnested, potential nonindependence was accounted for by using the TYPE = COMPLEX function in Mplus. Measurement (ie, configural, metric, and scalar) and structural (ie, factor variance and factor mean) invariance across sex were tested and assessed on the basis of Chen et al's guidelines.[39] Structural equation modeling was used to evaluate both the measurement models and the hypothesized structural model. In the hypothesized structural model, impulsivity dimensions were modeled as latent variables, and movement behavior combinations and the delay-discounting task were modeled as observed variables. Covariates (ie, sex, BMI, family income, parental education, and race and ethnicity) were included in the model to account for their potential effect on dimensions of impulsivity. Information regarding how the covariates were categorized is described in Table 1. Various fit indices were used to assess the measurement models, including the comparative fit index (CFI), standardized root square mean residual (SRMR), and root mean square error of approximation (RMSEA). Model fit was deemed acceptable if CFI values were >0.90 and if SRMR and RMSEA values were <0.08.[40] Composite reliability estimates[41] of latent variables were also computed. Statistical inferences were based on *P* values <.05 and confidence intervals (CIs).

Participants were classified into 1 of 8 possible movement behavior recommendation combinations: only PA, only ST, only sleep, PA + ST, PA + sleep, ST + sleep, PA + ST + sleep, and none (no recommendation met).

TABLE 2 Proportions of Study Variables

Descriptives	*N*	%
Sex		
Male	2152	47.6
Female	2372	52.4
Race and ethnicity		
Asian American	115	2.5
African American	452	10.0
White	2660	58.8
Hispanic	740	16.4
Multiracial	557	12.3
Movement behavior combinations		
Only PA	251	5.5
Only ST	522	11.5
Only sleep	1073	23.7
PA + ST	115	2.5
PA + sleep	212	4.7
ST + sleep	802	17.7
PA + ST + sleep	216	4.8
None	1333	29.4
Cash choice task		
Smaller, sooner	1841	40.7
Larger, later	2617	57.8
"Can't decide"	66	1.5

Participants were coded as 0 if they did not meet the behavior recommendation and as 1 if they did meet the behavior recommendation. The cash choice task was also dummy coded, wherein children who selected the larger, later reward or the "can't decide" option were coded as 0 and those who selected the smaller, sooner reward were coded as 1.

RESULTS

Descriptive Statistics and Measurement Models

Descriptive statistics are presented in Tables 1 and 2. Approximately 30% of the sample did not meet any of the recommendations, whereas only 4.8% of the sample met all movement behavior recommendations. Slight modifications were made to both measurement models (ie, deletion of negative factor loadings). The final UPPS-P solution comprised a 3-factor model (positive urgency, negative urgency, and perseverance), which showed excellent model fit ($\chi^2[51]$ = 329.58, $P < .001$, CFI = 0.97; SRMR = 0.03; RMSEA = 0.04 [90% CI: 0.031 to 0.038]). The 4-factor solution for the BIS/BAS Scale also revealed excellent model fit ($\chi^2[146]$ = 1415.86, $P <$ .001, CFI = 0.92; SRMR = 0.04; RMSEA = 0.04 [90% CI: 0.042 to 0.046]). Model fit for the measurement and structural invariance testing indicated acceptable model fit, and all changes in fit indices fell within acceptable ranges, as suggested by Chen et al[39] (see Supplemental Table 6).

Structural Model

UPPS-P

Meeting all movement behavior combinations (versus meeting none of the recommendations) was negatively related to positive and negative urgency and positively related to perseverance. Meeting the ST + sleep recommendations (versus meeting no recommendation) was most strongly associated with negative urgency (β = −.15), and meeting all movement behavior recommendations was most strongly associated with perseverance (β = .12). Compared with meeting no recommendation, meeting only the ST recommendation (β = −.08), the PA + ST recommendations (β = −.06), the ST + sleep recommendations (β = −.12), and all recommendations (β = −.09) were negatively associated with positive urgency. Meeting the ST + sleep ecommendations had the strongest association with positive urgency. Standardized β coefficients, SEs, *P* values, and CIs are presented in Table 3.

BIS/BAS

Apart from 3 exceptions (meeting only the sleep recommendation, only the PA recommendation, and the PA + ST recommendations), meeting all movement behavior combinations (versus meeting no recommendation) was negatively related to the BIS. Meeting the ST + sleep recommendations had the strongest relationship with the BIS (β = −.09). Meeting only the ST recommendation (β = −.08) and the ST + sleep recommendations (β = −.10) (versus meeting no recommendation) were negatively associated with BAS drive, with the latter combination having the strongest association with BAS drive. Meeting only the ST recommendation (β = −.07) and the ST + sleep recommendations (β = −.11) (versus meeting no recommendation) were negatively related to BAS fun, with the later combination having the strongest association. Meeting only the ST recommendation (β = −.04) and the ST + sleep recommendations (β = −.09) (versus meeting no recommendation) were negatively associated with BAS reward responsiveness. Meeting the PA + sleep recommendations (versus meeting no recommendation) was positively associated with BAS reward responsiveness (β = .05), and meeting only the PA recommendation (versus meeting no recommendation) was positively associated with BAS drive (β = .08), BAS fun (β = .09), and BAS reward responsiveness (β = .06). Standardized β coefficients, SEs, *P* values, and CIs are presented in Table 4.

Delay-Discounting Task

Compared with meeting no recommendation, participants meeting the sleep + PA recommendations (odds ratio [OR] = 0.74), the sleep + ST recommendations (OR = 0.81), and all recommendations (OR = 0.74) were less likely to select the smaller, sooner reward than the larger, later reward or the "can't decide" option. ORs, SEs, *P* values, and CIs are presented in Table 5.

DISCUSSION

The purpose of the current study was to determine if meeting the 24-hour movement behavior recommendations was associated with dimensions of impulsivity. In our results, it was shown that adherence to individual movement behavior recommendations as well as combinations of adherence to movement behavior recommendations were associated with each dimension of impulsivity. More specifically, children who met the sleep and ST recommendations scored favorably on all 8 dimensions of impulsivity (negative urgency, positive urgency, [lack of] perseverance, BIS, BAS drive, BAS reward, BAS fun-seeking, and delay-discounting) than children who did not meet any recommendation. In most cases, meeting the sleep + ST recommendations had the strongest association with the impulsivity dimensions. Although meeting all 24-hour movement behavior recommendations was associated with reduced impulsivity on 5 of the 8 domains (positive urgency, negative urgency, perseverance, BIS, delay-discounting), this movement behavior combination emerged as having the strongest association with only 1 of the impulsivity domains. Thus, with our results, it is suggested that meeting the PA recommendation provided no incremental predictive value beyond meeting the sleep + ST guidelines. The models explained 3.4% to 9.7% of the variance of impulsivity scores.

The sleep + ST movement behavior combination had the strongest association with most of the impulsivity measures (7 out of 8 dimensions), whereas the sleep + ST + PA behavior combination had the strongest association with perseverance. The former finding is not surprising, given that increased ST and reduced sleep have been independently associated with domains reflecting higher impulsivity among university students.[12,15] Moreover, more ST (eg, television, computers, video games, and mobile devices) is adversely associated with various sleep outcomes in school-aged children and adolescents, such as delayed bedtimes and shorter sleep duration.[42,43] Reduced ST has also been associated with greater sleep duration.[44] Our findings highlight that sleep and ST interact in a fashion that provides unique benefits compared with meeting either movement behavior alone and may be especially clinically relevant to target concurrently in interventions, given a small percentage of children meet these movement behavior guidelines.

Some possible mechanisms linking poor sleep and high amounts of ST with greater impulsivity are provided, with insights from basic science research. Reduced sleep duration may negatively impact impulsivity via its adverse biological effects on brain function and structure[45] and often leads to daytime sleepiness, which is associated with diminished inhibitory control and executive function processes and also predisposes youth to substance abuse and suicidality.[46] Modern forms of digital media (eg, excessive social media, video gaming) are highly reinforcing and have been shown to elicit responses in brain reward pathways that are similar to palatable foods[47] and drugs of abuse,[14] with associated decrements

TABLE 3 Standardized Path Coefficients Between Movement Behavior Recommendation Combinations and UPPS-P Dimensions

Path	β	SE	*P*	95% CI	R^2, %
Positive urgency					6.7
24-h movement combinations					
Only PA	.01	0.02	.638	−0.03 to 0.04	
Only ST[a]	−.08	0.02	<.001	−0.12 to −0.04	
Only sleep	−.01	0.02	.543	−0.05 to 0.03	
PA + ST[a]	−.06	0.01	<.001	−0.09 to −0.03	
PA + sleep	−.00	0.01	.944	−0.03 to 0.03	
ST + sleep[a]	−.12	0.02	<.001	−0.16 to −0.08	
PA + ST + sleep[a]	−.09	0.02	<.001	−0.12 to −0.05	
Covariates					
Female (reference: male)[a]	.07	0.02	.001	0.03 to 0.11	
BMI	.01	0.02	.559	−0.02 to 0.04	
Family income[a]	−.06	0.02	.002	−0.10 to −0.02	
Parent education[a]	−.07	0.02	.001	−0.12 to −0.03	
Ethnicity (reference: Asian American)					
White[a]	−.12	0.04	.003	−0.20 to −0.04	
African American	−.01	0.03	.668	−0.07 to 0.04	
Hispanic[a]	−.10	0.03	.001	−0.17 to −0.05	
Multiracial	−.04	0.03	.224	−0.11 to 0.03	
Negative urgency					4.0
24-h movement combinations[a]					
Only PA	−.04	0.02	.029	−0.08 to −0.00	
Only ST	−.13	0.02	<.001	−0.17 to −0.08	
Only sleep	−.06	0.02	.010	−0.11 to −0.01	
PA + ST	−.05	0.02	.002	−0.08 to −0.02	
PA + sleep	−.04	0.02	.033	−0.08 to −0.00	
ST + sleep	−.15	0.02	<.001	−0.20 to −0.10	
PA + ST + sleep	−.11	0.02	<.001	−0.14 to −0.08	
Covariate					
Female (reference: male)[a]	.09	0.02	<.001	0.05 to 0.12	
BMI	−.03	0.02	.093	−0.06 to 0.00	
Family income	.00	0.03	.958	−0.07 to 0.07	
Parent education	−.03	0.02	.304	−0.07 to 0.02	
Ethnicity (reference: Asian American)					
White	−.02	0.05	.649	−0.13 to 0.08	
African American	−.02	0.05	.705	−0.11 to 0.07	
Hispanic	−.05	0.05	.282	−0.15 to 0.04	
Multiracial	−.01	0.04	.763	−0.09 to 0.07	
Perseverance					4.0
24-h movement combinations[a]					
Only PA	.05	0.02	.001	0.02 to 0.08	
Only ST	.10	0.02	<.001	0.06 to 0.14	
Only sleep	.04	0.02	.023	0.01 to 0.07	
PA + ST	.09	0.01	<.001	0.06 to 0.12	
PA + sleep	.07	0.01	<.001	0.04 to 0.09	
ST + sleep	.10	0.02	<.001	0.06 to 0.15	
PA + ST + sleep	.12	0.02	<.001	0.09 to 0.15	
Covariates					
Female (reference: male)[a]	−.07	0.02	<.001	−0.11 to −0.04	
BMI	.01	0.02	.657	−0.03 to 0.05	
Family income[a]	.08	0.04	.030	0.01 to 0.15	
Parent education	−.03	0.02	.234	−0.07 to 0.02	
Ethnicity (reference: Asian American)					
White	.05	0.05	.370	−0.06 to 0.15	
African American[a]	.12	0.04	.002	0.04 to 0.19	
Hispanic[a]	.11	0.04	.004	0.03 to 0.19	
Multiracial	.06	0.04	.111	−0.01 to 0.14	

CIs are standardized.

[a] Indicates a significant path coefficient.

TABLE 4 Standardized Path Coefficients Between Movement Behavior Recommendation Combinations and BIS/BAS Dimensions

Path	β	SE	*P*	95% CI	R^2, %
BIS					
24-h movement combinations					3.4
Only PA	.00	0.02	.892	−0.04 to 0.04	
Only ST[a]	−.05	0.03	.045	−0.10 to −0.00	
Only sleep	−.00	0.03	.882	−0.06 to 0.05	
PA + ST	−.03	0.02	.076	−0.06 to 0.01	
PA + sleep[a]	−.04	0.02	.029	−0.07 to −0.00	
ST + sleep[a]	−.09	0.03	.002	−0.15 to −0.03	
PA + ST + sleep[a]	−.05	0.02	.006	−0.08 to −0.01	
Covariates					
Female (reference: male)[a]	−.01	0.02	<.001	−0.13 to −0.06	
BMI[a]	.04	0.02	.028	0.00 to 0.08	
Family income	.01	0.02	.714	−0.04 to 0.06	
Parent education[a]	−.06	0.02	.014	−0.10 to −0.01	
Ethnicity (reference: Asian American)					
White[a]	−.17	0.05	.002	−0.27 to −0.06	
African American[a]	−.09	0.04	.013	−0.16 to −0.02	
Hispanic	−.08	0.06	.156	−0.19 to 0.03	
Multiracial[a]	−.09	0.04	.030	−0.16 to −0.01	
BAS reward responsiveness					5.0
24-h movement combinations					
Only PA[a]	.06	0.02	.001	0.02 to 0.09	
Only ST[a]	−.04	0.02	.036	−0.08 to −0.00	
Only sleep	.00	0.02	.938	−0.04 to 0.04	
PA + ST	−.01	0.02	.653	−0.05 to 0.03	
PA + sleep[a]	.05	0.02	.002	0.02 to 0.08	
ST + sleep[a]	−.09	0.02	<.001	−0.04 to −0.05	
PA + ST + sleep	−.02	−0.01	.205	−0.10 to 0.00	
Covariates					
Female (reference: male)[a]	−.05	0.02	.018	0.01 to 0.10	
BMI[a]	.05	0.02	.001	0.02 to 0.09	
Family income[a]	−.05	0.02	.032	−0.02 to −0.00	
Parent education	.01	0.03	.963	−0.05 to 0.05	
Ethnicity (reference: Asian American)					
White	−.01	0.05	.905	−0.12 to 0.10	
African American[a]	.08	0.03	.009	0.02 to 0.14	
Hispanic	.05	0.05	.316	−0.05 to 0.14	
Multiracial	.02	0.04	.583	−0.05 to 0.10	
BAS drive					9.7
24-h movement combinations					
Only PA[a]	.08	0.02	<.001	0.05 to 0.11	
Only ST[a]	−.08	0.02	<.001	−0.11 to −0.05	
Only sleep	−.01	0.02	.338	−0.04 to 0.02	
PA + ST	.00	0.01	.900	−0.02 to 0.03	
PA + sleep	.04	0.02	.060	−0.00 to 0.09	
ST + sleep[a]	−.10	0.02	<.001	−0.14 to −0.06	
PA + ST + sleep	−.02	0.02	.243	−0.05 to 0.02	
Covariates					
Female (reference: male)[a]	−.09	0.01	<.001	0.07 to 0.12	
BMI[a]	.03	0.02	.026	0.00 to 0.06	
Family income[a]	−.08	0.03	.002	−0.14 to −0.03	
Parent education	−.03	0.02	.133	−0.07 to 0.00	
Ethnicity (reference: Asian American)					
White	−.04	0.04	.398	−0.12 to 0.05	
African American[a]	.09	0.03	.011	0.02 to 0.15	
Hispanic	.07	0.04	.102	−0.01 to 0.16	
Multiracial	.01	0.03	.676	−0.05 to 0.07	
BAS fun-seeking					5.0
24-h movement combinations					
Only PA[a]	.09	0.02	<.001	0.05 to 0.13	
Only ST[a]	−.07	0.02	.002	−0.11 to −0.02	

TABLE 4 Continued

Path	β	SE	*P*	95% CI	R^2, %
Only sleep	−.01	0.02	.578	−0.05 to 0.03	
PA + ST	.01	0.02	.753	−0.03 to 0.04	
PA + sleep	.04	0.02	.118	−0.00 to 0.08	
ST + sleep[a]	−.11	0.02	<.001	−0.15 to −0.07	
PA + ST + sleep	.01	0.02	.533	−0.03 to 0.05	
Covariates					
Female (reference: male)[a]	−.05	0.02	.014	0.01 to 0.10	
BMI	.03	0.02	.213	−0.02 to 0.07	
Family income	−.02	0.03	.363	−0.07 to 0.03	
Parent education	−.02	0.03	.366	−0.07 to 0.03	
Ethnicity (reference: Asian American)					
White	.11	0.06	.068	−0.01 to 0.23	
African American[a]	.12	0.05	.014	0.02 to 0.21	
Hispanic[a]	.11	0.05	.026	0.01 to 0.20	
Multiracial[a]	.09	0.04	.022	0.01 to 0.16	

CIs are standardized.
[a] Indicates a significant path coefficient.

in attention, cognitive control, and impulsivity.[14] These neurobiological correlates of excessive ST, combined with a prominent dynamic inherent in many screen-based technologies that necessitate immediate responding while punishing delayed responses, may serve to reinforce impulsivity and undermine the development of self-regulatory abilities.

Meeting the PA recommendation (either alone or in combination with meeting the sleep recommendation) was positively related to BAS reward responsiveness and BAS drive. This finding is somewhat consistent with previous research, indicating that greater levels of PA are linked with higher scores on BAS drive[48] and that greater PA enjoyment is positively associated with BAS reward responsiveness.[49] We also found that PA was associated with lower negative urgency and positively associated with perseverance. These novel findings are generally consistent with a recent systematic review in which it was shown that PA is associated with improved executive functioning in youth.[17] The inconsistent associations observed may reflect differences in PA dose, measurement, and sample characteristics across studies. Clearly, more research is needed to determine how PA alone or combined with other movement behavior recommendations is associated with children's impulsive traits. The prospective, longitudinal measures from the ABCD Study will be

TABLE 5 Relationships Between Movement Behavior Recommendation Combinations and Delay-Discounting Task

Path	OR	SE	*P*	95% CI
Smaller, sooner (reference: larger, later and "can't decide" option)				
24-h movement combinations				
Only PA	1.00	0.12	.972	0.79 to 1.26
Only ST	1.00	0.13	.971	0.79 to 1.29
Only sleep	0.96	0.07	.557	0.83 to 1.11
PA + ST	0.84	0.16	.274	0.58 to 1.23
PA + sleep[a]	0.74	0.08	.001	0.60 to 0.92
ST + sleep[a]	0.81	0.07	.005	0.68 to 0.97
PA + ST + sleep[a]	0.74	0.09	.003	0.57 to 0.94
Covariates				
Female (reference: male)[a]	1.16	0.07	.027	1.03 to 1.31
BMI	0.97	0.02	.211	0.93 to 1.02
Family income[a]	1.06	0.03	.012	1.02 to 1.11
Parent education[a]	0.92	0.03	.001	0.87 to 0.97
Ethnicity (reference: Asian)				
White	0.81	0.14	.185	0.57 to 1.15
African American	0.87	0.17	.456	0.60 to 1.28
Hispanic	1.16	0.26	.536	0.75 to 1.81
Multiracial	0.77	0.12	.063	0.56 to 1.06

[a] Indicates a significant path coefficient.

important to better dissect these relationships.

There are limitations and strengths to our study. First, with respect to limitations, our results are based on cross-sectional data, preventing us from drawing any causal inferences regarding associations. Future researchers should not only conduct longitudinal studies but also explore the bidirectional link between the movement behaviors and impulse control. That is, children with impulse control problems may spend more time on rewarding screens, may be more likely to procrastinate bedtime, and may engage in low levels of PA (because the health benefit in future is delayed), which in turn may exacerbate impulsivity, creating a vicious cycle. Second, a single item was used to measure PA, which may have played a role in the lack of observed findings between PA and dimensions of impulsivity. Using other measures of PA (eg, wearable devices) would help to improve the internal validity of our findings. Third, the screen-based questions in our study only assessed the amount of time spent in separate ST behaviors. Other characteristics of ST that can potentially affect young people's behaviors should also be considered. Such characteristics include screen content, timing exposure, size of screen, frequency of phone-checking, and simultaneous use of multiple screens.[43] The act of simultaneously using electronic devices (eg, mobile device, computer or tablet) while watching television is referred to as "screen-stacking" (also known as media multitasking) and is a trend expected to grow as screen-based technologies continue to rapidly evolve. In fact, in recent evidence, it has been shown that nearly half of evening television watchers engage in "screen-stacking."[50] Despite the acknowledged limitations, our study has notable strengths. In this study, we were the first to examine the concurrent associations between sleep, ST, and PA on impulsivity among children. Furthermore, our research is the first to include the UPPS-P and BIS/BAS in one model. By modeling different dimensions of impulsivity simultaneously, we were able to account for the interplay between these dimensions (via variance).

CONCLUSIONS

In the results of the current study, we showed that children who met the sleep + ST recommendations consistently reported lower levels of impulsivity compared with not meeting any movement behavior guidelines. Meeting all movement behavior recommendations was associated with reduced impulsivity on most but not all measures, suggesting that meeting the PA recommendation provided no incremental benefit in terms of reduced impulsivity, although PA is well documented to be important for physical and mental health in youth and should still be encouraged.[51] Our findings have important implications for pediatricians, psychiatrists, educators, parents, and policy makers as they suggest that strategies to limit recreational ST while simultaneously promoting early, routine bedtimes and more sleep may enhance the treatment and prevention of impulsivity-related psychiatric disorders.

ACKNOWLEDGMENTS

Data used in the preparation of this article were obtained from the ABCD Study (https://abcdstudy.org), held in the National Institute of Mental Health Data Archive. This is a multisite, longitudinal study designed to recruit more than 10 000 children aged 9 to 10 years and manage them over 10 years into early adulthood. A listing of participating sites and a complete listing of the study investigators can be found at https://abcdstudy.org/principal-investigators.html. ABCD Study consortium investigators designed and implemented the study and/or provided data but did not necessarily participate in the analysis or writing of this report. This article reflects the views of the authors and may not reflect the opinions or views of the National Institutes of Health or ABCD Study consortium investigators. The ABCD Study data repository grows and changes over time. The ABCD Study data used in this report came from National Institute of Mental Health data (DOI: 10.15154/1412097).

ABBREVIATIONS

ABCD: Adolescent Brain Cognitive Development
BAS: Behavioral Activation System
BIS: Behavioral Inhibition System
CFI: comparative fit index
CI: confidence interval
OR: odds ratio
PA: physical activity
RMSEA: root mean square error of approximation
SRMR: standardized root square mean residual
ST: screen time

PEDIATRICS (ISSN Numbers: Print, 0031-4005; Online, 1098-4275).

FINANCIAL DISCLOSURE: The authors have indicated they have no financial relationships relevant to this article to disclose.

FUNDING: The Adolescent Brain Cognitive Development Study is supported by the National Institutes of Health and additional federal partners under award numbers U01DA041022, U01DA041028, U01DA041048, U01DA041089, U01DA041106, U01DA041117, U01DA041120, U01DA041134, U01DA041148, U01DA041156, U01DA041174, U24DA041123, and U24DA041147. A full list of supporters is available at https://abcdstudy.org/nih-collaborators. Funded by the National Institutes of Health (NIH).

POTENTIAL CONFLICT OF INTEREST: The authors have indicated they have no potential conflicts of interest to disclose.

REFERENCES

1. Reynolds B, Ortengren A, Richards JB, de Wit H. Dimensions of impulsive behavior: personality and behavioral measures. *Pers Individ Dif.* 2006;40(2): 305–315
2. Miller M, Hinshaw SP. Attention-deficit/ hyperactivity disorder. In: *Encyclopedia of Mental Health.* 2nd ed. Amsterdam, The Netherlands: Elsevier; 2015:116–123
3. Perry JL, Carroll ME. The role of impulsive behavior in drug abuse. *Psychopharmacology (Berl).* 2008; 200(1):1–26
4. Shin SH, Chung Y, Jeon SM. Impulsivity and substance use in young adulthood. *Am J Addict.* 2013;22(1):39–45
5. Rømer Thomsen K, Callesen MB, Hesse M, et al. Impulsivity traits and addiction-related behaviors in youth. *J Behav Addict.* 2018;7(2):317–330
6. Waxman SE. A systematic review of impulsivity in eating disorders. *Eur Eat Disord Rev.* 2009;17(6):408–425
7. Miller JD, Zeichner A, Wilson LF. Personality correlates of aggression: evidence from measures of the five-factor model, UPPS model of impulsivity, and BIS/BAS. *J Interpers Violence.* 2012;27(14):2903–2919
8. Krueger RF, Markon KE, Patrick CJ, Benning SD, Kramer MD. Linking antisocial behavior, substance use, and personality: an integrative quantitative model of the adult externalizing spectrum. *J Abnorm Psychol.* 2007; 116(4):645–666
9. Maxfield BL, Pepper CM. Impulsivity and response latency in non-suicidal self-injury: the role of negative urgency in emotion regulation. *Psychiatr Q.* 2018; 89(2):417–426
10. Huang YH, Liu HC, Tsai FJ, et al. Correlation of impulsivity with self-harm and suicidal attempt: a community study of adolescents in Taiwan. *BMJ Open.* 2017;7(12):e017949
11. Matricciani L, Olds T, Petkov J. In search of lost sleep: secular trends in the sleep time of school-aged children and adolescents. *Sleep Med Rev.* 2012;16(3): 203–211
12. Miller MB, DiBello AM, Lust SA, Meisel MK, Carey KB. Impulsive personality traits and alcohol use: does sleeping help with thinking? *Psychol Addict Behav.* 2017;31(1):46–53
13. Abe T, Hagihara A, Nobutomo K. Sleep patterns and impulse control among Japanese junior high school students. *J Adolesc.* 2010;33(5):633–641
14. Weinstein A, Livny A, Weizman A. New developments in brain research of internet and gaming disorder. *Neurosci Biobehav Rev.* 2017;75:314–330
15. Wilmer HH, Chein JM. Mobile technology habits: patterns of association among device usage, intertemporal preference, impulse control, and reward sensitivity. *Psychon Bull Rev.* 2016;23(5):1607–1614
16. Minear M, Brasher F, McCurdy M, Lewis J, Younggren A. Working memory, fluid intelligence, and impulsiveness in heavy media multitaskers. *Psychon Bull Rev.* 2013;20(6):1274–1281
17. Donnelly JE, Hillman CH, Castelli D, et al. Physical activity, fitness, cognitive function, and academic achievement in children: a systematic review. *Med Sci Sports Exerc.* 2016;48(6):1197–1222
18. Diamond A. Executive functions. *Annu Rev Psychol.* 2013;64:135–168
19. Medina JA, Netto TL, Muszkat M, et al. Exercise impact on sustained attention of ADHD children, methylphenidate effects. *Atten Defic Hyperact Disord.* 2010;2(1):49–58
20. Smith AL, Hoza B, Linnea K, et al. Pilot physical activity intervention reduces severity of ADHD symptoms in young children. *J Atten Disord.* 2013;17(1): 70–82
21. CSEP SCPE. Canadian 24-hour movement guidelines: an integration of physical activity, sedentary behaviour, and sleep. Available at: https:// csepguidelines.ca/. Accessed July 24, 2019
22. Walsh JJ, Barnes JD, Cameron JD, et al. Associations between 24 hour movement behaviours and global cognition in US children: a cross-sectional observational study. *Lancet Child Adolesc Health.* 2018;2(11): 783–791
23. Roman-Viñas B, Chaput JP, Katzmarzyk PT, et al; ISCOLE Research Group. Proportion of children meeting recommendations for 24-hour movement guidelines and associations with adiposity in a 12-country study. *Int J Behav Nutr Phys Act.* 2016;13(1):123
24. Thivel D, Tremblay MS, Katzmarzyk PT, et al; ISCOLE Research Group. Associations between meeting combinations of 24-hour movement recommendations and dietary patterns of children: a 12-country study. *Prev Med.* 2019;118:159–165
25. Sampasa-Kanyinga H, Standage M, Tremblay MS, et al. Associations between meeting combinations of 24-h movement guidelines and health-related quality of life in children from 12 countries. *Public Health.* 2017;153: 16–24
26. Garavan H, Bartsch H, Conway K, et al. Recruiting the ABCD sample: design considerations and procedures. *Dev Cogn Neurosci.* 2018;32:16–22
27. Barch DM, Albaugh MD, Avenevoli S, et al. Demographic, physical and mental health assessments in the adolescent brain and cognitive development study: rationale and description. *Dev Cogn Neurosci.* 2018;32(32):55–66
28. Luciana M, Bjork JM, Nagel BJ, et al. Adolescent neurocognitive development and impacts of substance use: overview of the adolescent brain cognitive

development (ABCD) baseline neurocognition battery. *Dev Cogn Neurosci*. 2018;32(32):67–79

29. Bruni O, Ottaviano S, Guidetti V, et al. The Sleep Disturbance Scale for Children (SDSC). Construction and validation of an instrument to evaluate sleep disturbances in childhood and adolescence. *J Sleep Res*. 1996;5(4): 251–261
30. Sharif I, Wills TA, Sargent JD. Effect of visual media use on school performance: a prospective study. *J Adolesc Health*. 2010;46(1):52–61
31. Centers for Disease Control and Prevention. Youth risk behavior survey. 2016. Available at: https://www.cdc.gov/healthyyouth/data/yrbs/index.htm. Accessed July 17, 2019.
32. Scott JJ, Morgan PJ, Plotnikoff RC, Lubans DR. Reliability and validity of a single-item physical activity measure for adolescents. *J Paediatr Child Health*. 2015;51(8):787–793
33. Nascimento-Ferreira MV, Collese TS, de Moraes ACF, Rendo-Urteaga T, Moreno LA, Carvalho HB. Validity and reliability of sleep time questionnaires in children and adolescents: a systematic review and meta-analysis. *Sleep Med Rev*. 2016; 30:85–96
34. Zapolski TCB, Stairs AM, Settles RF, Combs JL, Smith GT. The measurement of dispositions to rash action in children. *Assessment*. 2010;17(1): 116–125
35. Pagliaccio D, Luking KR, Anokhin AP, et al. Revising the BIS/BAS Scale to study development: measurement invariance and normative effects of age and sex from childhood through adulthood. *Psychol Assess*. 2016;28(4): 429–442
36. Wulfert E, Block JA, Santa Ana E, Rodriguez ML, Colsman M. Delay of gratification: impulsive choices and problem behaviors in early and late adolescence. *J Pers*. 2002;70(4):533–552
37. Matusiewicz AK, Carter AE, Landes RD, Yi R. Statistical equivalence and test-retest reliability of delay and probability discounting using real and hypothetical rewards. *Behav Processes*. 2013;100:116–122
38. Muthén L, Muthén B. *Mplus User's Guide*. 8th ed. Los Angeles, CA: Muthén & Muthén; 2017
39. Chen FF, Hayes A, Carver CS, Laurenceau JP, Zhang Z. Modeling general and specific variance in multifaceted constructs: a comparison of the bifactor model to other approaches. *J Pers*. 2012;80(1):219–251
40. Marsh HW, Hau K-T, Grayson D. Goodness of fit in structural equation models. In: Maydeu-Olivares A, McArdle JJ, eds. *Contemporary Psychometrics: A Festschrift for Roderick P. McDonald*. Mahwah, NJ: Larence Erlbaum; 2005
41. Raykov T. Estimation of composite reliability for congeneric measures. *Appl Psychol Meas*. 1997;21(2):173–184
42. Cain N, Gradisar M. Electronic media use and sleep in school-aged children and adolescents: a review. *Sleep Med*. 2010;11(8):735–742
43. Hale L, Guan S. Screen time and sleep among school-aged children and adolescents: a systematic literature review. *Sleep Med Rev*. 2015;21:50–58
44. Calamaro CJ, Mason TBA, Ratcliffe SJ. Adolescents living the 24/7 lifestyle: effects of caffeine and technology on sleep duration and daytime functioning. *Pediatrics*. 2009;123(6). Available at: www.pediatrics.org/cgi/content/full/123/6/e1005
45. Taki Y, Hashizume H, Thyreau B, et al. Sleep duration during weekdays affects hippocampal gray matter volume in healthy children. *Neuroimage*. 2012; 60(1):471–475
46. Maski KP, Kothare SV. Sleep deprivation and neurobehavioral functioning in children. *Int J Psychophysiol*. 2013; 89(2):259–264
47. O'Donnell S, Epstein LH. Smartphones are more reinforcing than food for students. *Addict Behav*. 2019;90:124–133
48. Voigt DC, Dillard JP, Braddock KH, Anderson JW, Sopory P, Stephenson MT. Carver and White's (1994) BIS/BAS scales and their relationship to risky health behaviours. *Pers Individ Dif*. 2009;47(2):89–93
49. Schneider ML, Graham DJ. Personality, physical fitness, and affective response to exercise among adolescents. *Med Sci Sports Exerc*. 2009;41(4):947–955
50. Adam EK, Snell EK, Pendry P. Sleep timing and quantity in ecological and family context: a nationally representative time-diary study. *J Fam Psychol*. 2007;21(1):4–19
51. Biddle SJH, Asare M. Physical activity and mental health in children and adolescents: a review of reviews. *Br J Sports Med*. 2011;45(11):886–895

Social Media: Anticipatory Guidance

David L. Hill, MD*

*Department of Pediatrics, University of North Carolina School of Medicine, Chapel Hill, NC

Practice Gaps

Clinicians should be aware of roles that social media play in child and adolescent health and development and be prepared to guide parents and patients toward best practices in social media use.

Objectives

After completing this article, readers should be able to:

1. Recognize the major benefits and risks posed by social media throughout the course of child development.
2. Become comfortable addressing the roles that social media play in the most important aspects of child health and development, including psychosocial development, academic performance, healthy weight and sleep habits, and minimizing high-risk behaviors.

INTRODUCTION

Dr Victor Strasburger wrote in 2010: "The media are not the leading cause of any health problem in childhood or adolescence. However, they can make a substantial contribution to virtually every health concern that pediatricians and parents have about young people—aggression, sex, drugs, obesity, self-image and eating disorders, depression and suicide, even learning disorders and academic achievement." (1) Since that time, the use of digital media has proliferated, along with our understanding of how such media affect child and adolescent health and development. To Dr Strasburger's list we would now add risks including sleep deprivation, problematic Internet use, and Internet gaming disorder. At the same time, this assessment overlooks some of the potential benefits that social media have to contribute to children's education, connectedness, and resilience.

Although many pediatricians feel comfortable using some social media platforms, fewer counsel parents and patients on social media use. The American Academy of Pediatrics updated its media use guidelines for children and adolescents in 2016, (2)(3) but only 20% of parents of children aged 0 to 8 years report any familiarity with those guidelines. (4) Most tweens (children ages 8–12 years) (84%) and teens (66%) report that their parents have talked to them about the content of their media use, but 30% of teens also say that their parents have little to no knowledge of what they post on social media. (5) As pediatricians become increasingly aware of social determinants of health, we must remember that media use is among the most powerful influences on child well-being.

AUTHOR DISCLOSURE Dr Hill has disclosed that he is a member of the speaker's bureau for Chicco car seats, is a consultant for Gerber, is involved with social media efforts for the National Fisheries Institute and Evivo Probiotics, and serves on the scientific advisory board for Before Brands/ SpoonfulOne. This commentary does not contain a discussion of an unapproved/ investigative use of a commercial product/ device.

DEFINING SOCIAL MEDIA

Merriam-Webster Dictionary defines social media as "forms of electronic communication (such as websites for social networking and microblogging) through which users create online communities to share information, ideas, personal messages, and other content (such as videos)." (6) In the past, social media were largely restricted to dedicated platforms such as Facebook and Instagram, but "social" is increasingly cropping up in unexpected places. Online games such as Minecraft and Fortnight allow for real-time communication and interaction among players. Gamers can also broadcast their play and interact with fans on sites such as Twitch.

YouTube serves up an endless stream of videos, but it also allows users to comment, post, and form groups around interests or content producers. Fitness trackers such as MapMyRun are an example of gamification; they allow users to share their results, compete with each other across time and space, and comment on each other's performance. Even toys for small children such as Webkinz come with a social media component that is often more important than the physical object. In this fast-moving field, the only reliable constant is the guarantee that most of the previous examples will seem dated in a very short time.

SOCIAL MEDIA USE BY 0- TO 8-YEAR-OLDS

According to Common Sense Media's latest survey in 2017, most children now access social media through mobile devices such as smartphones and tablets. (4) Ninety-eight percent of children ages 0 to 8 years now live in a home with some sort of mobile device, and 42% of these children own their own tablets. Children in this age group spend an average of 45 minutes a day on mobile devices, but social media account for less than half of that time, approximately 25 minutes a day. Young children have little interest in adult social media sites, preferring "social games" targeted at their demographic, such as Club Penguin, Animal Jam, and Minecraft.

Among the youngest children, ages 0 to 2 years, pediatricians might feel heartened that the average time spent on screens has dropped from 58 minutes a day to 42 minutes, with the caveat that this reduction is not statistically significant. Most children's exposure to social media at this age comes via their parents' involvement, through postings of photographs, videos, and blogs ("sharenting"). (7) Concerns about these postings center on the permanent "digital footprint" that they leave online, long before children can consent to any use of their personal information. In 1 study, 56% of parents were deemed to have posted "potentially embarrassing" information about their young children online, information that may be accessible to children's future peers, the public, and predators. (8)

As recently as 2017, only 20% of parents of children ages 0 to 8 years reported familiarity with the American Academy of Pediatrics screen use guidelines. (4) Familiarity with the guidelines increased with household income and white race, with a corresponding decrease in early childhood screen use.

SOCIAL MEDIA USE BY 8- TO 12-YEAR-OLDS

No observer will be surprised to learn that children's media use takes a dramatic jump between ages 8 and 12 years, to an average of 6 hours a day. (5) This alarming figure, however, obscures the broad range of media habits that these children actually display. Because many children are using more than 1 platform or device at a time, it does not mean that they are sitting in front of screens for a solid 6 hours daily but that the aggregate of all digital media use adds up to that time over 24 hours. Six percent of these children use no electronic media, and, at the other end of the spectrum, 11% use for more than 8 hours daily. More than a quarter (28%) use for less than 2 hours daily.

Children spend little of this time on dedicated social media platforms; passive programming ("TV") and video gaming dominate their screen time. Social media time grows, however, with 58% of youth using social media daily by age 13 years for an average of 2 hours a day. Girls are much more likely to spend time on social platforms than are boys, who still prefer gaming.

SOCIAL MEDIA USE BY TEENS

Smartphones have transformed the media landscape for teens, with 95% reporting access to a smartphone and 45% saying they are online "almost constantly." (9) Social media platforms still attract more girls than boys, and boys still edge out girls in the world of gaming, but only by a slim margin (97% vs 83%). Preferred social media platforms vary by race, sex, and socioeconomic status. As of 2018, Facebook use was in decline among teens, with YouTube, Instagram, and Snapchat ascendant as the top 3 teen platforms.

Teens display varying and balanced views regarding the impact of social media on their well-being. Forty-five percent feel that social media have a neutral effect on well-being, 31% report a positive effect, and 24% think that the effect is mostly negative. Those who favor social media point to the platforms' ability to connect them to friends and family, provide current news and information, and help them find others with similar interests. Detractors cite bullying and gossip, unrealistic social comparisons, and distraction from real-life friendships as key drawbacks of social media use.

UTILITY OF ANTICIPATORY GUIDANCE

Evidence suggests that time spent exploring social media use during child and teen wellness visits has a measurable and positive effect on outcomes. (10) Overall, increased parental monitoring reduces children's and teens' risky health behaviors, and parents who talk to their kids about media use better understand what their children are watching and posting. (11)

Social media can be more difficult for parents to monitor than gaming and passive viewing: 84% of pre-teenagers (ages 8–12 years) said that their parents have talked with them about the content of media they use, but only 54% thought that their parents knew "a lot" about their social media use. (12) Parents give a similar consensus: 82% of parents reported "high awareness" of the content their child sees on television, 56% reported high awareness of online video content, and only 40% reported high awareness of social media exposures. (13)

POTENTIAL HARMS OF SOCIAL MEDIA FOR CHILDREN AGES 0 TO 5 YEARS

Infants, toddlers, and young children learn best from personal interactions with the adults closest to them. Counseling on social media in this age group, then, starts with parents' and caregivers' media use. Parents distracted by their own social media use tend to demonstrate fewer interactions with their children, both verbal and nonverbal. (14) They may display poor responsiveness to their children's needs, resulting in increased conflict as children act out in frustration. (15)

Although not specific to social media, other screen media contribute significantly to childhood obesity, starting at a young age. (16) These effects are mediated more by advertising of unhealthy foods and diminished satiety cues than by decreased total daily activity. (17) Although most research data on media use and obesity come from studies on television, the social games favored by younger children allow for copious advertising integrated into their content, promoting unhealthy nutrition, and building brand loyalty among the youngest consumers.

Burgeoning literature ties exposure to digital media/screens to sleep disruption even as pediatricians are becoming increasingly aware of the critical role that healthy sleep plays in children's physical, mental, and developmental health. Although many parents might see digital media as a sleep aid, the presence of a screen in the bedroom leads to fewer minutes of sleep for children at all ages, including infants. (18) Stimulating media content can certainly lead to psychomotor excitement and sleep interruption, but the more pervasive mechanism of sleep disruption seems to be the effect of blue-enriched light on melatonin secretion from the pineal gland. (2) Even the most calming content, if viewed on electronic screens, can affect melatonin secretion and disrupt healthy sleep patterns.

Although social media have not been specifically implicated as negatively affecting young children's intellectual and social development, screen media as a whole have negatively affected child development, either actively or by displacing other activities that contribute more to mental and physical health. (2) Excessive television viewing in young children has been correlated with delays in cognition, language acquisition, and social-emotional development. The risks increase with earlier initiation of viewing, greater hours of total use, and less educational content. Face-to-face communication and real-world interactions are critical for optimal development. Co-viewing and higher educational content can mitigate some of the negative effects.

POTENTIAL BENEFITS OF SOCIAL MEDIA FOR CHILDREN AGES 0 TO 5 YEARS

Electronic media, including educational television programming and well-designed mobile applications, do contribute to learning in children ages 3 to 5 years, with some preliminary studies possibly extending this threshold down to 15 months of age. (2) The extent to which these data apply specifically to social media will depend on how well these platforms integrate features critical to learning, such as interactivity and scaffolding (the ability of a program to build on previously attained skills). Overall, there remains a large gap between the number of applications and programs that claim to support early childhood learning and those whose claims are backed by evidence.

ANTICIPATORY GUIDANCE FOR PARENTS OF CHILDREN AGES 0 TO 5 YEARS

What, then, can pediatricians suggest to parents of young children regarding the use of social media? Suggestions include the following:

- Avoid media use in children younger than 18 to 24 months except for video chatting alongside a parent or caregiver.
- For children 18 to 24 months and beyond, use the American Academy of Pediatrics Family Media Use

Plan to determine the optimal balance of healthy activities and use of digital media. Limit displacement of healthy activities by excessive digital media use.

- For children 18 to 24 months, choose high-quality programming, referring to resources such as Common Sense Media and Sesame Workshop for guidance. Co-view and co-participate.
- For children 2 to 5 years of age, limit screen time to 1 hour per day. Ensure adequate physical activity, sleep, face-to-face communication, conversations, device-free meals, etc. Choose evidence-based, high-quality programming. Co-view/engage. Avoid violent and fast-paced content. Turn off devices when not in use. Avoid using media as a calming tool—discuss alternatives during the visit. Monitor content, test apps out first. Establish media-free zones (1 hour before bedtime, meal times, and parent-child talk and play time). (2)
- At all ages parents should limit their own electronic media use in the presence of children to increase engagement and learning opportunities.

POTENTIAL HARMS OF SOCIAL MEDIA FOR OLDER CHILDREN AND ADOLESCENTS

The relationship between traditional media use and childhood and adult obesity is among the best-demonstrated harmful effects of excessive media use. (3) Bedroom television, unhealthy snacking behavior, and exposure to advertising all seem to play a role. Available studies, however, do not demonstrate a relationship between social media use and unhealthy weight. (19)

Sleep disruption remains a significant and well-demonstrated concern in this age group. (20) Factors exacerbating the effect include the presence of mobile devices in the bedroom and the use of social media specifically; the resulting poor sleep correlates with poorer school performance in affected children. (3)

Many psychologists diagnose and treat the closely related conditions of problematic Internet use and Internet gaming disorder. Although the World Health Organization recently proposed that Internet gaming disorder be included in the *International Classification of Diseases, 11th Revision*, the most recent edition of the American Psychiatric Association's *Diagnostic and Statistical Manual of Mental Disorders* stops short of giving these conditions an official designation, suggesting instead that researchers further investigate the extent to which these conditions result directly from screen media use or are mere manifestations of underlying psychiatric disorders such as anxiety and depression. (21)

Both disorders present with similar symptoms: preoccupation with the activity, decreased interest in offline or "real-life" relationships, unsuccessful attempts to decrease use, and withdrawal symptoms on reducing use of electronic media. Estimates put the prevalence of both disorders in the ballpark of 8% for youth ages 8 to 18 years. (3) The Personal Internet Gaming Disorder Evaluation-9 is a specific tool for diagnosing gaming disorder. (22) Top instruments for screening for problematic Internet use include the Internet Addiction Test, the Young of the Internet Addiction Questionnaire, the Chen Internet Addiction Scale, and the Internet Addiction Scale. (23)

Psychologists also continue to debate the role that social media play in the development of anxiety and depression. Researchers have long demonstrated a strong correlation between excessive social media use and mood disorders, (24)(25) but whether the relationship is causal remains unclear. (26) The association may rest in part on how different people use social media. Those who follow friends seem less depressed than those who follow strangers, (27) and users who post actively seem happier than those who "lurk," preferring to view others' posts. (28)

Although multiple studies have demonstrated a possible relationship between digital media use and symptoms of attention-deficit/hyperactivity disorder, none has determined that media actually cause the condition. (29) Media multitasking, however, does negatively affect attention and focus. Half of all teens report that they "often" or "sometimes" watch TV (51%) or use social media (50%) while doing homework. More say they text (60%) and listen to music (76%). (5) Although most teens do not believe that these behaviors affect the quality of their work, extensive data suggest otherwise. (30)

Social media potentially expose children and adolescents to "cyberbullying." Between 10% and 40% of children report an experience with cyberbullying. Compared with in-person bullying, however, it is much less clear online who is the bully and who is the victim, with the roles often alternating over the course of an exchange. (31) Other features that distinguish cyberbullying include that the perpetrator can be anonymous, the bullying can invade the home and other normally safe spaces, the bullying can occur at any time of day, and the bullying can spread rapidly to large numbers of witnesses. As with traditional bullying, cyberbullying may lead to long- and short-term negative social, academic, and health consequences for both parties.

Extensive data tie traditional media use to high-risk behaviors in teens. Increased exposure to such behaviors in television shows and movies puts teens at risk for tobacco use, alcohol abuse, drug abuse, and high-risk sexual practices. The literature supporting such a correlation to social media is less robust, but adolescents who engage in these behaviors often reference them in their social media posts. Pediatricians treating eating disorders should also be aware of a whole genre of "pro-ana" sites offering "thinspiration" to sufferers who may be looking for more positive feedback for restrictive eating than they receive from friends and family members. (3)

"Sexting" refers to the electronic transmission of nude or seminude images as well as sexually explicit text messages. Between 10% and 12% of youth ages 10 to 19 years report sending or receiving a sext. Girls especially report feeling pressured into sending a sext. Sexting in and of itself may be seen as a normal part of how teens explore their sexuality, but it can also serve as a marker for higher-risk sexual behaviors. (32) Sexts do not always remain private; they can be shared widely and can be difficult or impossible to remove from the Internet. The greatest risk of sexting may involve the unforeseen legal consequences in states where sexting by minors is defined as a form of child pornography.

Social media may also facilitate online sexual solicitation of minors by strangers. The best estimate is that 9% of youth aged 10 to 17 years have been subject to online solicitation, and 4% of these children and teens report that the solicitor attempted to arrange a face-to-face encounter. In these cases most solicitors were honest about their identities and their intentions rather than posing as other people. (33)(34)

POTENTIAL BENEFITS OF SOCIAL MEDIA FOR OLDER CHILDREN AND ADOLESCENTS

Young people increasingly integrate social media into their daily lives as a venue through which they can accomplish the developmental tasks of adolescence: identity development, aspirational development, and peer engagement. Researchers have identified associations between teen social media use and increased self-esteem, increased social capital (resources accessed through one's social relationships), safe identity exploration, development of social supports, and opportunities for self-disclosure. (35) Teens can test different identities and attitudes online and obtain instantaneous feedback from peers and strangers alike.

Social media also expose youth to new ideas and information and help raise awareness of current events and issues. Teens may turn to social media as a set of tools to enhance community participation and civic engagement or to collaborate on academic and community projects. Social media also provide a natural and convenient platform for maintaining and building relationships with friends and family members who may not be physically accessible. (3) Young people who feel marginalized often use social media to connect with sympathetic networks and share their experiences to reduce feelings of isolation. (36)

Social media can provide uniquely flexible and accessible platforms for promoting healthy behaviors. Examples abound of support networks built around chronic conditions such as diabetes and asthma. (37) Young people often start online when seeking answers to their health-related questions. (38) Pediatricians eager to enhance wellness among their patients and their communities can leverage the power of social media to teach digital literacy and help promote reliable sources of health information.

ANTICIPATORY GUIDANCE FOR SCHOOL-AGE CHILDREN AND ADOLESCENTS (3)

Pediatricians can also do or advise the following during well-care encounters with school-age children, adolescents, and caregivers:

- Promote adherence to healthy sleep, exercise, academic, and social habits using the American Academy of Pediatrics Family Media Use Plan (www.HealthyChildren.org/MediaUsePlan)
- Consider using screening tools for problematic Internet use and Internet gaming disorder (the Internet Addiction Test, the Young of the Internet Addiction Questionnaire, the Chen Internet Addiction Scale, and the Internet Addiction Scale) when appropriate
- Encourage families to place appropriate limits on media to mitigate negative effects and avoid displacement of healthier activities
- Total hours per day—use the Family Media Use Plan to promote healthy choices
- Type of media—encourage active engagement rather than passive viewing
- Discourage media use during homework outside of what is needed to complete the assignment; consider placing devices in a central location so that parents can monitor that use is for schoolwork
- Protect bedtime
- No digital media/screens for 1 hour before sleep
- No devices in rooms after bedtime
- Tech-savvy parents may be encouraged to use restrictive devices and apps to limit Internet access based on content or time of day
- Encourage families to designate media-free meal times (dinner) and zones (bedrooms)
- Remind families to keep other caregivers (grandparents, babysitters) aware of expectations and rules

- Encourage families to select and co-view media with their children, with a focus on family and community engagement
- Encourage families to have ongoing communication with children about online citizenship and safety
- Treating others with respect online and offline
- Avoiding cyberbullying and sexting
- Being wary of online solicitation and reporting any suspicious contacts
- Avoiding communications that can compromise personal privacy and safety
- Remind children to actively develop a network of trusted adults who can engage with children through social media and to whom children can turn when they encounter challenges
- Encourage parents to use resources on digital literacy such as those found at Common Sense Media (www.commonsense.org) to help educate children and teens on media use
- Encourage parents to model the digital behavior they expect from their children and teens

Summary

- Social media have become ubiquitous in the lives of children, adolescents, and their parents, with significant effects on child health, development, and well-being.
- Based on some research evidence (11)(12) as well as consensus, (2)(3) pediatricians should address social media use with parents at every stage of childhood and adolescent development.
- Based on some research evidence as well as consensus, (2)(3) limiting electronic media use, including social media use, can improve childhood health behaviors around sleep, obesity, attention, intellectual and social development, and high-risk behaviors.
- Based on some research evidence as well as consensus, (2)(3) pediatricians can work with parents to optimize children's and teens' social media use for positive outcomes, including learning, community involvement, improved health behaviors, social and emotional development, and connection to family members, communities, and friends. Parents can help children by monitoring their social media activity, co-viewing or co-participating in media use, setting appropriate limits, serving as role models for media use and digital citizenship, and building an awareness of risks around digital presentation.

References for this article are available at https://doi.org/10.1542/pir.2018-0236.

ARTICLE

The Health Effects of Video Games in Children and Adolescents

Daniel Alanko, MD*

*Hasbro Children's Hospital and Alpert School of Medicine at Brown University, Providence, Rhode, Island

PRACTICE/EDUCATION GAPS

During the past several decades, video games have played an ever-larger role in the lives of children; however, quality research on the health effects of video game use has lagged. Recent high-quality studies have refined our understanding of this association. Clinicians should have a basic understanding of the effects of video game use on the health of children and adolescents and should be able to guide patients and caregivers on appropriate use. With the recent addition of gaming disorder to the *International Classification of Diseases, 11th Revision,* clinicians should know how to identify and screen for pathologic gaming.

OBJECTIVES *After completing this article, readers should be able to:*

1. Identify the major benefits and risks of video game use on child health and development.
2. List the symptoms of the *International Classification of Diseases, 11th Revision*'s newly added gaming disorder and distinguish between healthy and pathologic gaming.
3. Gain comfort in addressing the role that video games play on physical, cognitive, mental, and social health when engaging with patients and their caregivers.

ABSTRACT

Play has always been an essential part of childhood, but it looks different for modern children, who increasingly engage in virtual play. More than 90% of children older than 2 years play video games, and three-quarters of American households own a video game console. Children 8 to 17 years of age spend an average of 1.5 to 2 hours daily playing video games. Recent developments framed by decades of research have provided insight into how games influence children's physical health, mental health, social behaviors, and cognitive development. Anticipatory guidance surrounding media use is often centered on screen time, but pediatricians should have some knowledge of the unique benefits and risks associated with this nearly ubiquitous activity. In light of the recent addition of gaming disorder

AUTHOR DISCLOSURE: Dr Alanko has disclosed no financial relationships relevant to this article. Dr Alanko's current affiliation is Department of Pediatric Emergency Medicine at Newark Beth Israel Medical Center, Newark, New Jersey. This commentary does not contain a discussion of an unapproved/investigative use of a commercial product/device.

ABBREVIATIONS

AAP	American Academy of Pediatrics
ADHD	attention-deficit/hyperactivity disorder
APA	American Psychological Association
ESRB	Entertainment Software Rating Board
GADIS	Gaming Disorder Scale
ICD-11	*International Classification of Diseases, 11th Revision*
IGDT-10	Ten-Item Internet Gaming Disorder Test

to the *International Classification of Diseases, 11th Revision*, this review includes a discussion of the epidemiology, clinical features, and diagnosis of gaming disorder, including the use of existing screening tools. As games become more popular while ever-increasing in scope and complexity, this review aims to educate the modern pediatric provider about what is known, what is uncertain, and how to use this knowledge in the management of both healthy and unhealthy video gaming in children.

INTRODUCTION

During the past few decades, video games have become a favorite pastime for many children, and their use continues to increase. (1) The percentage of American children who play video games is estimated to be more than 90%, increasing to 97% among those ages 12 to 17 years. (2) In 2021, the average 8- to 12-year-old played approximately 1.5 hours of video games daily, and the average 13- to 17-year-old played for almost 2 hours. (3) Video games occupy a significant portion of children's days, making them a potential driver of child health and development in both positive and negative ways. As researchers find new connections between gameplay and well-being, it is important for pediatricians to have some familiarity with the effects of this almost-ubiquitous activity. Several articles in the past few years have reviewed the literature surrounding screen time and social media use in children. (4)(5)(6) This review summarizes the expansive topic of childhood video game use and its unique implications for health and development with the purpose of pediatrician education. Some facets of this topic are politicized and highly debated, with parents, researchers, game producers, and policy makers having different, sometimes competing, opinions. (7) However, high-quality research during the past decade has clarified our understanding of some of these effects. Note that most research in children has focused on adolescents, with less robust literature on preadolescents. In addition, some of the research discussed in this article was performed in adults and is discussed if relevant in the absence of reliable studies in children.

THE IMPACT OF VIDEO GAMES ON PHYSICAL HEALTH

Researchers have long known about the adverse effects that screen time can have on child and adolescent health. The relationship between excessive screen time and obesity itself is well-documented. (8) Spending time in front of screens has the potential to increase BMI by several mechanisms, including increased sedentary time, increased snacking and decreased satiety cues, disrupted sleep, and exposure to food marketing. (9) Although the data on media use such as television and video viewing is clear, data are more mixed for video games. A 2020 review found 26 articles concerning the association between video games and obesity. (10) The authors concluded that there was inconsistent evidence of the relationship between video games and obesity, with 14 articles finding no association and 12 articles finding a positive association between video game use and weight gain. Compared with resting in a sitting position, gaming increases heart rate, blood pressure, and overall caloric expenditure. (11) However, this is likely mitigated by findings in several studies that video gamers consume more snacks, more fatty foods, and more sugary beverages than nongamers. (11)(12)(13) Gamers are exposed to less food and product promotion than traditional media, although mobile phone and tablet games frequently contain advertisements. Overall, the association between playing video games and obesity is less clear than for more passive media use such as television viewing, but the net effect is likely a slight tendency toward weight gain and unhealthy eating.

This does not include newer physically active games, or "exergames," which have shown promise in promoting a range of healthier behaviors. (10) One example most people have heard of is *Pokémon Go*, a game that relies on the player's movement through the real world via walking or running to progress. By coupling exercise (something children should do) with an appealing activity such as achievement in a video game (something children want to do), enjoyment of the less-preferable activity is increased. As of 2019, players of *Pokémon Go* had walked an astounding 14 billion miles catching and hatching the small animated creatures known as Pokémon. (14) A 2021 systematic review found that playing *Pokémon Go* had measurable positive effects on physical, mental, and social health. (15) There are many exergames now available, from *Pokémon Go* to the ever-popular *Dance Dance Revolution* series to newer, accessible virtual reality systems; all have the potential to increase activity in previously sedentary patients. When used regularly, exergames have been shown to have beneficial effects for weight loss, exercise program adherence, and even depression. (16)(17)(18)

It is also known that the use of screens close to bedtime decreases both quantity and quality of sleep. Playing video games in the evening is associated with longer time to fall asleep, decreased total sleep, and architectural changes in rapid eye movement and slow-wave sleep in children. There may also be an association between playing games in the evening and next-day attention and memory. These effects may be mediated by several mechanisms, including disruption of normal melatonin secretion due to light exposure, psychomotor stimulation by more exciting games, or displacement of sleep by gameplay. (19)(20)(21)(22) Several small studies have found that playing fast-paced, violent games and playing for a prolonged period (>2.5 hours) are associated with significant disruptions in sleep compared with shorter, more relaxed gameplay. (23)(24) Sleep deprivation has been associated with a multitude of undesirable health effects, including decreased executive functioning skills and academic performance, irritability and mood disorders, and physical inactivity. (25) Having a screen in the child's bedroom, in addition to effects on sleep, decreases parents' ability to monitor gaming activities and has been shown independently to be linked to obesity and to decreased academic performance. (26)(27)

THE IMPACT OF VIDEO GAMES ON COGNITIVE DEVELOPMENT

Physical play has distinct advantages over virtual play, including the development of fine and gross motor skills and reduced screen time. Young children show deficits in learning from screens compared with direct interaction with other humans. (28) The dangers of excess media use in young children are well-known, and the benefits of hands-on play cannot be understated. (4)

Not all screen time is equal, and the active attention and participation asked of the player make video games more cognitively stimulating than television watching. Virtual play cannot replace physical play, although there is some value in solving puzzles and overcoming obstacles even through a screen. There is experimental evidence in older children and adolescents that consistent video gameplay can enhance a variety of cognitive domains, including problem solving, working memory, information processing, and flexibility. (29) Action games may improve visual processing and reaction times. (30)(31)(32) Puzzle games, memory games, and strategy games may improve other aspects of executive functioning. (33)(34)(35) Much like playing a sport, playing video games strengthens connections through repetition. There is evidence that some of these skills transfer to the real world, as a small study found that training with action games improved reading abilities in children with dyslexia. (36)

The ability of games to promote cognitive development depends on the context of the gaming and the age of the child. Many principles from the American Academy of Pediatrics' (AAP's) Media and Young Minds 2016 policy statement can be applied to video game use. (4) Parents should monitor children's gaming activities, keep video games away from eating and sleeping spaces, and avoid fast-paced and violent games in young children. When possible, games should be enjoyed together to promote learning. For example, open-ended games such as *Minecraft* and *Roblox* are great for encouraging creativity, but as with physical play, learners may derive the greatest benefit when co-playing with an adult who can provide direction, context, and opportunity for socialization. The most recent screen time guidelines from the AAP recommend against most screen use for children younger than 2 years; this should apply to video games as well. Children between 3 and 5 years of age should be limited to 1 hour per day of media use, including video games.

Limit setting is important for school-age children and adolescents as well, and more liberal gameplay time must be balanced with other essential needs. Families should create and consistently follow plans for video game use that ensure adequate sleep (8–12 hours nightly depending on age), physical activity (1 hour daily), time for schoolwork, and in-person interaction with family and friends. (37) Sensible limits on gaming may be different between children depending on their ability to meet these needs.

The relationship between video game use and attention problems has been much studied. A 2018 systematic review found a statistically small relationship between screen media use and attention-deficit/hyperactivity disorder (ADHD)–related behaviors. (38) This association is theorized to be stronger for video games than traditional media due to higher levels of engagement and arousal. Most studies have been cross-sectional, making causation difficult to establish. A recent longitudinal study did find that video game use predicted ADHD symptoms in adolescents, but existing ADHD symptoms did not predict future video game use, suggesting a causal link. (39) Children with ADHD are also more likely to use video games excessively, with longer play times on average and more addictive behavior. (40)(41) Therefore, children with ADHD and their guardians may benefit from education about appropriate play, particularly limit setting to ensure that video games do not interfere with other necessary activities.

THE IMPACT OF VIDEO GAMES ON MENTAL HEALTH

The link between gaming and mental health is complex. The overall effect on emotional well-being seems to be related to many factors, including time spent gaming, motivations for gaming, and whether gaming is done alone or socially. Many studies have found associations between excessive gameplay and negative psychosocial outcomes. (42) "Excessive play" is used generally to represent a state of addiction that affects other aspects of a player's life, which will be discussed more later. People who engage in moderate video game use have improved affective symptoms compared with those who play video games excessively or not at all. (43)(44) One study in college-age men found that they played more video games when stressed, lonely, or bored, without significant effects on BMI or grade point average, suggesting a healthy means of socialization and relaxation. (45) A variety of commercial video games have shown efficacy in reducing stress and anxiety in both adolescents and young adults, even with brief play sessions. (46) In 1 study, gamers cited feelings of stress relief, reduced anxiety, and a "sense of purpose" from accomplishment in games. (1) In addition to the amount of gameplay, motivations for gameplay are important. Playing for enjoyment or for social purposes improves psychological symptoms compared with playing purely for escapism or achievement. (47) Overall, playing video games can have positive effects on children's mental health, but they must be enjoyed in a healthy way. This is to say that one must consider not only the amount of time spent playing but also why they are playing the game and whether they are truly enjoying their experience.

Video games also offer a way for children to explore new identities. For example, a child assigned a certain gender at birth can play a video game as a character with a different gender expression. They can then explore this identity in an environment that they may consider safer. Some games even offer romantic relationships with characters of the same sex, which can offer a unique opportunity to LGBTQ adolescents who may not be ready or able to express their sexuality in the real world.

The potential for negative psychological effects must be considered as well. A central question of gaming research during the past 4 decades has been whether violent video games can make children more aggressive. This issue is often at the forefront of media and policy maker discussions about video games, and it came to a head in the late 1990s and early 2000s after a string of mass shootings and the popularity of the *Grand Theft Auto* series, with the first title being banned in Britain, Germany, and France due to its "extreme violence." A violent game is one that allows players to kill or inflict serious harm against human or humanlike characters. This definition is broad and applies to games depicting intense violence, blood, and gore such as the *Grand Theft Auto* and *Call of Duty* series. (48) It can also apply to more child-friendly games such as *Minecraft*, which has a content warning for "fantasy violence," and *Fortnite*, which contains violence but not blood and gore. Video-game content warnings and age ratings will be discussed more later herein.

Several meta-analyses have found a significant relationship between violence in video games and aggressive behavior in players. (49)(50) In their 2020 updated resolution on the topic, the American Psychological Association (APA) does recognize a link between violent video games and increased aggression (using insults, making threats, yelling, pushing), decreased sensitization, and decreased empathy but not actual violence or criminal behavior. (51) This report has come under criticism from some experts. One 3-year-long longitudinal study found that violent video games had no effect on aggression when controlling for other factors, such as depression, exposure to family and peer violence, and antisocial personality traits. (52) There are concerns about publication bias; more recent studies with preregistered hypotheses have found weaker associations between violent video games and aggressive behavior than previous work. Despite the controversy, the APA maintains that this association has been shown consistently over time. The style of game seems to matter, as self-reports of aggression have been shown in several studies to be lower when playing video games with social aspects such as multiplayer games with cooperative play. (53)(54) Postgame aggression may also be influenced by the context in which the violence occurs, as players enacting violence through a moral character (against "bad" people) experienced lower levels of aggression than players enacting violence through an immoral character (against "good" or "innocent" people). (55)(56) More quality studies are needed to further explore this relationship. Enough evidence exists to suggest that playing violent video games can contribute to aggression, but the APA resolution states that "attributing violence to violent video gaming is not scientifically sound and draws attention away from other factors [which contribute to violence]."

Video games also have a strong potential for addiction. For many, they offer a tempting escape from real life, along with engaging design and satisfying reward systems. Problems arise when players game excessively and compulsively. Proposed symptoms of gaming disorder (or Internet gaming disorder) lean heavily on criteria for substance use disorder and include a preoccupation with games, mood symptoms such as irritability and sadness when the game is taken away (withdrawal), increasing amounts of time spent gaming (tolerance), and unsuccessful attempts to quit. (57) The *International Classification of Diseases, 11th Revision* (*ICD-11*), which is published by the World Health Organization and took effect on January 1, 2022, includes gaming disorder for the first time, and the *Diagnostic and Statistical Manual of Mental Disorders, Fifth Edition* (published by the APA in 2013) includes Internet gaming disorder simply as a "condition for further study." (58) The *ICD-11* requires "marked distress or significant impairment in personal, family, social, educational or occupational functioning" for gaming disorder to be diagnosed. Gaming disorder is a type of behavioral addiction and can be compared clinically to gambling disorder. There remains a lack of consensus on the assessment and symptoms of problematic gaming, making prevalence estimates difficult. (59) A recent study of more than 100,000 gamers found that approximtely 2% had disordered gaming behavior when assessed with the new World Health Organization framework. (60) The best estimates of prevalence among adolescents are even higher at 3.3% to 4.6%, with boys affected at a rate of 5:1 compared with girls. (61)(62) Problematic gaming behavior is more prevalent in male adolescents and those with ADHD, and other coexisting disorders such as depression and anxiety should be considered. (40)(63)(64)

Providers should be aware of gaming disorder as an entity, and at the same time should be thoughtful about assigning the diagnosis and referring to treatment. False-positive cases in healthy gamers can cause tensions in the parent-child relationship, inappropriate treatment, and stigma. The association between time spent gaming and severity of disordered gaming behavior is not perfectly linear, and someone who plays for 30 hours per week may have a healthier relationship with video games than someone who plays for 20 hours per week. (60) Patients meeting the criteria for gaming disorder play for an average of 35 to 40 hours per week. Treatment centers have been established in some East Asian countries, (65) but at this time patients in the United States should be referred to cognitive behavioral therapy or family therapy services with the understanding that there is a lack of randomized controlled research concerning the efficacy of treatment options. (66)(67) In-office strategies such as motivational interviewing and Screening, Brief Intervention, and Referral to Treatment may also be used. There currently exist several screening tools for gaming disorder that have been validated in preliminary studies, examples of which are the Ten-Item Internet Gaming Disorder Test (IGDT-10) and the Gaming Disorder Scale (GADIS), with versions for adolescents and for parents. (68)(69)(70) The IGDT-10 is based on the Diagnostic and Statistical Manual of Mental Disorders, Fifth Edition framework, and the GADIS is based on the *ICD-11* framework. The IGDT-10 can be administered more rapidly and has a simpler scoring system. Advantages of the GADIS include a stronger emphasis on negative consequences and availability of a caregiver questionnaire for patients who may have unreliable self-ratings. A version of the GADIS was also developed specifically for adolescents (ages 10–17 years). Both are screening tools and should be used in conjunction with clinical interviews for diagnosis. The questions contained in the English versions of both tools can be found in Tables 1 and 2.

THE IMPACT OF VIDEO GAMES ON SOCIAL HEALTH

In our increasingly digital, globalized world we rely on technology to stay close to people. This shift has accelerated during the past 2 years during the coronavirus disease 2019 pandemic, with more people using social media and online video games to communicate with friends and family. (1) Many children use video games as a tool to build and maintain relationships with their peers. A 2021 online poll found that more than half of teens prefer video games as a way to keep in touch with friends over video calling or social media. (71) Cooperating in a game environment to achieve

Table 1. Ten-Item Internet Gaming Disorder Test

In the past 12 months:
1. When you were not playing, how often have you fantasized about gaming, thought of previous gaming sessions, and/or anticipated the next game?
2. How often have you felt restless, irritable, anxious, and/or sad when you were unable to play or played less than usual?
3. Have you ever felt the need to play more often or played for longer periods to feel that you have played enough?
4. Have you ever unsuccessfully tried to reduce the time spent on gaming?
5. Have you ever played games rather than meet your friends or participate in hobbies and pastimes that you used to enjoy before?
6. Have you played a lot despite negative consequences (eg, losing sleep, not being able to do well in school or work, having arguments with your family or friends, and/or neglecting important duties)?
7. Have you tried to keep your family, friends, or other important people from knowing how much you were gaming or have you lied to them regarding your gaming?
8. Have you played to relieve a negative mood (eg, helplessness, guilt, or anxiety)?
9. Have you risked or lost a significant relationship because of gaming?
10. Have you ever jeopardized your school or work performance because of gaming?

Answer choices include never, sometimes, or often. If at least 5 criteria are met (with answers of "often"), the screen is considered positive. Of note, items 9 and 10 belong to the same criterion, and a positive response on either or both counts as 1 criterion met.
Reprinted with permission from Orsolya Király, PhD, Institute of Psychology, ELTE Eötvös Loránd University, Budapest, Hungary.

Table 2. Gaming Disorder Scale for Adolescents

In the past 12 months:

1. I often play games more frequently and longer than I planned to or agreed upon with my parents.
2. I often cannot stop gaming even though it would be sensible to do so or, for example, my parents have told me to stop.
3. I often do not pursue interests outside the digital world because I prefer gaming. For example, I do not meet with friends/my partner in real life, do not attend sports clubs/societies, do not read books or make music because of gaming.
4. I neglect daily duties, because I prefer gaming. Daily duties include, for example, doing grocery shopping, cleaning, tidying up after myself, tidying up my room, fulfilling obligations for school/apprenticeship/job.
5. I continue gaming even though it causes me stress with others. This means, for example, stress with my parents, siblings, friends, partner, or teachers because of gaming.
6. I continue gaming although it harms my performance at school (or apprenticeship/job). For example, I'm late, I do not participate in class, I neglect homework, and I get worse grades because of gaming.
7. Due to gaming, I neglect my appearance, personal hygiene, and/or my health. For instance, I sleep less, eat unhealthy, and/or exercise less because of gaming.
8. Due to gaming, I risk losing important contacts or have lost them already. This includes contacts with partners, friends, acquaintances, or family.
9. Due to gaming, I have disadvantages at school/apprenticeship/job. For example, I got bad (final) grades, I'm unable to continue to next grade or do not graduate, I have no place for training or studying, and/or I got a poor reference or a warning/dismissal as a result of gaming.
10. In the past year, how often did you experience the conflicts or difficulties described in the statements 1 to 9 due to gaming? (not at all, single days, longer periods, or almost daily)
    Original scale includes 3 additional questions further clarifying item 10

Items 1 through 9 are Likert-type responses ranging from strongly disagree to strongly agree. If positive for both cognitive behavioral symptoms (items 1, 2, 4, and 5) and negative consequences (items 3, 6, 7, 8, and 9) and the time criterion is met (item 10), then the screen is indicative of gaming disorder.

Reprinted with permission from Kerstin Paschke, MD, Center for Psychosocial Medicine, German Center for Addiction Research in Childhood and Adolescence, University Medical Center Hamburg-Eppendorf, Hamburg, Germany.

objectives can be more stimulating than other forms of online socialization. In the *Journal of Cyberpsychology, Behavior, and Social Networking,* psychologist Brenda Wiederhold compared this "virtual meeting place" to a mall or a playground during prepandemic times. (72) As more traditional types of in-person play became less feasible, children engaged in more social gaming with friends and family to fill the gap. Online video games provide an accessible tool that can help children meet their social needs. Playing video games with friends may be a normal part of social development for today's children, just as playing tag on the playground was for previous generations.

Compared with playing alone, being socially active in games has been associated with lower levels of depression and addiction even in those who play heavily. (63) Other benefits include increased prosocial behaviors such as cooperation and empathy, and decreased aggression after playing violent video games with social components. (53)(73)(74)(75) There are clear benefits to playing with others, and cooperative play (working with others toward a common objective) has emotional and social advantages over competitive play (trying to defeat others). (76) There is no strong evidence that certain levels of gaming negatively affect family closeness, activity involvement, or school engagement. (44) However, online games should not completely replace in-person interaction; 1 study found that social connections were strongest when friends had both online and offline interaction. (77) Families can also benefit from playing video games together. Parents who take an active interest in their child's gaming have more opportunities for co-play, which has known social and developmental benefits over playing alone. (78)

Social gaming exists in many forms. It can be 2 people playing together in the same room, which is known as "couch co-op," or it can be 2 people far from each other who have never met. Social video games can also serve more specific roles. Cooperation in games can help build social behaviors that may be difficult to develop for some children in real life, such as those with autism spectrum disorder, social anxiety, or other socialization disorders/avoidant behaviors. People who have trouble finding friends in real life can find others with shared interest in a game.

Types of social video games and popular examples are as follows:

- Cooperative games (playing with others): *Minecraft, Animal Crossing, Stardew Valley, Farming Simulator* series, *Lego* series, *Overcooked* series, *Cuphead*
- Competitive games (playing against others): *Super Smash Bros.* series, *Mario Kart* series, *Mario Party* series, *Wii Sports, Fall Guys, Rec Room*
- Cooperative and competitive elements (can play with others and against others): *Roblox, Rocket League, Among*

Us, *Pokémon series, Fortnite*, Overwatch*, League of Legends*, Sea of Thieves*, Valorant*, Apex Legends*, Call of Duty* series*, *Halo* series*

- Massive multiplayer online role-playing games (cooperative and competitive elements): *MapleStory, Wizard101, World of Warcraft*, RuneScape*, Sea of Thieves*, The Elder Scrolls Online**
- Socialization/chat games: *VRChat*, Second Life*, Avakin Life**

*These games contain content that may not be appropriate for children younger than 13 years.

CYBERBULLYING IN VIDEO GAMES

Online experiences with other real players do have the potential for more harmful interactions. Although traditionally more of an issue on social media platforms, cyberbullying also exists in online video games. According to the Centers for Disease Control and Prevention (CDC), more than 15% of high school students report being bullied online in the past year, and cyberbullying (similar to traditional bullying) can have negative psychological and social effects. (79)(80) Cyberbullying has been associated with higher rates of depression and suicidality, social isolation, and difficulty trusting peers. Bullying in online games takes several forms: exclusion from playing with others, targeting a single player and intentionally causing them to lose the game, and verbal harassment, which can range from generally offensive language to personal attacks to bigoted slurs targeting sexuality, race, or gender.

Cyberbullying in games can come from people the victim knows or does not know in real life, can be completely anonymous due to aliases, can occur at any time of day, and can invade safe spaces at home that in-person bullying cannot. Certain video games are infamous for having a "toxic" player community; that is, one that is more exclusionary and less friendly, and other games have friendlier communities. (81) In addition to cyberbullying, online multiplayer games have the potential to expose children to strangers with malicious intent who could exploit younger players sexually or financially.

The 2011 AAP report on "The Impact of Social Media on Children, Adolescents, and Families" provides recommendations around Internet safety and cyberbullying. Several actions are recommended for pediatricians, including encouraging parents to talk with their children about online use and active participation in monitoring their child's online activities. Parents should know who their children are playing with, and children should be educated about online safety, including what bullying looks like. Cyberbullying in online games is harder to track than on social media because there is often no record of conversations or of in-game activities. Parents with children younger than 13 years should be more vigilant, including keeping gaming devices in family areas and encouraging children to play without headphones. Older adolescents may want more privacy while gaming with peers, but parents should engage them in regular conversation about their experiences. Many online games have processes for reporting and banning players who engage in inappropriate behavior. Certain kinds of behavior should be reported to the child's school or to the authorities in the case of criminal behavior.

HOW PARENTS CAN MAKE GAMES SAFER

As discussed, it is beneficial for parents to take an interested and active role in their child's video gaming because this can strengthen family connections, enrich learning, and make games safer. It is also important because children, particularly preadolescents, lack the ability to contextualize mature gaming content. Games may include violence, strong language, or suggestive themes such as substance use, gambling, and sexual content. Younger children may have trouble enjoying these games in a safe way, leading to problems with personal development and socialization. (82) In addition to these adult themes, female representation in video games remains a problem. As is the case with media in general, female characters in games are frequently subject to subordination to male characters, objectification, and hypersexualization. With repeated exposure, this can lead to sexist beliefs in men and low self-efficacy and self-objectification in women. (83) A caregiver can help by being present while the child plays to give context about fictitious depictions compared with real-life social expectations, and the importance of respect and consent.

In addition to this more active role, there exist tools to help parents make informed decisions about which games their children are exposed to. The Entertainment Software Rating Board (ESRB) is a self-regulatory organization established by the video game industry in 1994 to assign content ratings to all consumer video games in the United States. The 3-part rating system informs parents about age-appropriateness, specific content warnings, and interactive elements such as communication with others online, sharing location data, or in-game purchases. (48) The ESRB has several ratings: E (everyone), all ages; E 10+ (everyone 10+), everyone older than 10 years; T (teen), everyone older than 13 years; M (mature), everyone older than 17 years; and Ao (adults only), everyone older than 18 years.

This is the most widely used rating system for commercially available games, and parents should be aware of this system and how to use it. However, independent game creators do not necessarily need to have a rating assigned to their game to sell it, particularly on mobile phone and tablet platforms, so awareness of game content is still important. Most gaming devices now come with parental control features, and even those with cursory knowledge of technology can set restrictions on mature content, unauthorized purchases, and the ability to communicate online with others. In addition to official rating bodies such as the ESRB, websites such as commonsensemedia.org and askaboutgames.com offer parent-focused reviews and ratings to help in determining appropriateness.

ACKNOWLEDGMENT

Special acknowledgment to Dr Allison Heinly, who helped with editing this manuscript and with citation management software. Dr Heinly specializes in pediatric primary care and is an assistant professor of pediatrics at the Alpert School of Medicine at Brown University.

Summary

- Video games have become a major part of many children's lives, and their use has significant effects on various aspects of health and well-being. They can be a normal part of modern childhood development and recreation when used in a healthy way.
- Providers and parents should use recommendations from the American Academy of Pediatrics concerning media use, such as setting consistent limits based on the child's age and ensuring that gaming does not interfere with adequate physical activity, sleep, and other behaviors essential to health (https://www.aap.org/en/patient-care/media-and-children/policies-on-children-and-media and healthychildren.org).
- Based on some research evidence, playing video games is a risk factor for obesity. Based on some research evidence, physically active video games (exergames) can be an effective weight loss tool for some patients.
- Based on some research evidence, playing video games in the evening reduces sleep quality and quantity. Providers should stress the importance of playing early and of removing screens from bedrooms.
- Based on some research evidence, video games can reduce anxiety and stress when enjoyed in moderation. In addition, playing with others provides mental health benefits compared with playing games alone.
- Based on some research evidence and consensus, violent video games should be considered a risk factor for increased aggressive behavior. However, the effect is likely influenced by other risk factors for aggression, and no clear link with actual violence has been demonstrated.
- Based on some research evidence and consensus, gaming disorder is a discrete diagnosis added to the *International Classification of Diseases, 11th Revision* describing addictive behavior around video game use. Providers should be able to identify potentially problematic gaming, which shares features with substance use disorders (preoccupation, withdrawal, tolerance, etc). Male adolescents and those with attention-deficit/hyperactivity disorder are at increased risk. Formal screening with a validated screening tool and referral to cognitive behavioral therapy are potential next steps.
- Online multiplayer games can expose children to cyberbullying, which can have adverse effects on mental health, and to strangers with unknown intent. Parents should know who their child is interacting with online and should educate their children about online citizenship and safety.
- Providers should encourage parents to look at Entertainment Software Rating Board ratings or a similar rating system before purchasing video games for their children to determine whether the game is age- and content-appropriate. Co-play with caregivers should be encouraged because it can strengthen family connections, make games safer, and help children derive the greatest developmental benefits from their play.

References and teaching slides for this article can be found at https://doi.org/10.1542/pir.2022-005666.

Childhood and Adolescent Television Viewing and Metabolic Syndrome in Mid-Adulthood

Nathan MacDonell, BBiomedSc, Robert J. Hancox, MD

abstract

BACKGROUND: Excessive sedentary behaviors, such as television viewing or other screen time, may have adverse metabolic effects. We hypothesized that television viewing time in childhood would be associated with the risk of metabolic syndrome at 45 years of age.

METHODS: We studied a population-based birth cohort born in Dunedin, New Zealand in 1972 and 1973. Parent- and self-reported weekday television viewing times were recorded at ages 5, 7, 9, 11, 13, 15, and 32 years. The primary outcome was metabolic syndrome at age 45 years, defined as 3 or more of: high glycated hemoglobin; high waist circumference; high blood triglyceride; low high-density lipoprotein cholesterol; and high blood pressure. Reported television viewing time and metabolic syndrome data were available for 870 (87%) of 997 surviving participants.

RESULTS: Mean television viewing time between ages 5 and 15 years was associated with metabolic syndrome at 45 years of age. This association persisted after adjusting for sex, socioeconomic status, and BMI at age 5 (odds ratio: 1.30; 95% confidence interval: 1.08 to 1.58; $P = .006$) and after further adjustment for adult television viewing (odds ratio: 1.26; 95% confidence interval: 1.03 to 1.54; $P = .026$). Childhood television viewing was also associated with lower cardiorespiratory fitness and higher BMI at 45 years of age.

CONCLUSIONS: Time spent watching television during childhood and adolescence is associated with the risk of metabolic syndrome in mid-adulthood. Interventions to reduce screen time for children and young people may have long-lasting benefits for health.

Department of Preventive and Social Medicine, Dunedin School of Medicine, University of Otago, Dunedin, New Zealand

Mr MacDonnell wrote the first draft of the manuscript, conceived and designed the analysis, and interpreted the data; Dr Hancox conceived and designed the analysis, interpreted the data, and critically reviewed and revised the manuscript; and both authors approved the final manuscript as submitted and agree to be accountable for all aspects of the work.

DOI: https://doi.org/10.1542/peds.2022-060768

Accepted for publication May 9, 2023

Address correspondence to R.J. Hancox, MD, Department of Preventive and Social Medicine, Dunedin School of Medicine, University of Otago, PO Box 56, Dunedin 9054, New Zealand. E-mail: bob.hancox@otago.ac.nz

PEDIATRICS (ISSN Numbers: Print, 0031-4005; Online, 1098-4275).

FUNDING: The Dunedin Multidisciplinary Health and Development Research Unit is funded by the Health Research Council of New Zealand (program grant 16-604) and has also received funding from the New Zealand Ministry of Business, Innovation and Employment. This research was also supported by UK MRC grant MR/P005918/1 and US-National Institute of Aging grants R01AG032282 and R01AG069936. Nathan McDonnell was supported by an Otago Medical Research Foundation Middlemass Family Summer Scholarship. Robert Hancox received no additional funding. The funder/sponsor did not participate in the work.

(Continued)

WHAT'S KNOWN ON THIS SUBJECT: Sedentary behavior is associated with the risk of metabolic syndrome, obesity, and poor fitness. There is some evidence that this risk may extend from childhood into adulthood, but long-term follow-up studies are lacking.

WHAT THIS STUDY ADDS: Television viewing in childhood and adolescence is associated with a higher risk for metabolic syndrome, obesity, and poor fitness in mid-adulthood. This association is independent of adult viewing, indicating that childhood television viewing has long-term adverse effects on metabolic health.

To cite: MacDonell N, Hancox RJ. Childhood and Adolescent Television Viewing and Metabolic Syndrome in Mid-Adulthood. *Pediatrics.* 2023;152(2):e2022060768

ARTICLE

Sedentary behaviors, such as television viewing, increase the risk of morbidity and mortality.[1-3] Young people now spend much more time undertaking sedentary behaviors than previous generations, a trend that accelerated during the coronavirus disease 2019 pandemic.[4-7] The long-term consequences of this are not yet clear.

The Dunedin Multidisciplinary Health and Development Study (Dunedin study) previously reported that childhood and adolescent (ages 5–15 years) television viewing was predictive of several indicators of poor health, including higher BMI and lower cardiorespiratory fitness (oxygen consumption at maximal exertion [$V'O_2$ max]) at ages 26 and 32 years.[8,9] In addition, television viewing time from childhood and adolescence was a better predictor of both BMI and cardiorespiratory fitness at age 32 than concurrent viewing,[9] suggesting that childhood television viewing has lasting effects on adult health, regardless of changes in habits in adulthood.[1,2,9,10]

Metabolic syndrome is a cluster of cardiometabolic risk factors associated with the risk of type 2 diabetes mellitus, cardiovascular disease, and nearly 60% higher mortality.[11-13] Metabolic syndrome can be defined in several ways, but the core features include obesity, insulin resistance or hyperglycemia, hypertension, and dyslipidemia.[11,14] The worldwide prevalence of metabolic syndrome has increased along with aging populations and the prevalence of obesity. These secular trends also parallel increases in sedentary behavior (particularly screen time) and reductions in physical activity.[13] Few long-term studies have investigated whether television viewing in childhood increases the risk for metabolic syndrome: most research has either been cross-sectional or is limited by short follow-up times.[15-17] One study found that watching "several shows a day" compared with "one show/week or less" at age 16 was associated with metabolic syndrome at age 43 years. This association remained after adjustment for adult television and other potential confounders.[2] Increasing television viewing over 6 to 12 years follow-up of Danish adolescents was associated with metabolic syndrome scores and insulin levels independently of physical activity,[18] while digital media use by European children was associated with metabolic syndrome, independently of physical activity, over 6 years follow-up.[19] The Nurses' Health Study II identified an association between television viewing at ages 3 to 5 years and 5 to 10 years and adult type 2 diabetes in women.[20] More than 4 hours per day of screen time at age 16 in the 1970 British Birth Cohort was associated with the risk of developing type 2 diabetes over the following 30 years.[21] Television viewing at age 23 was also associated with adverse cardiometabolic profiles at age 44 years in the 1958 British Birth Cohort, but this was not significant after adjusting for early adult BMI, suggesting that the critical risk period for developing metabolic syndrome due to sedentary behavior may be in childhood or adolescence.[22]

We tested the hypothesis that sedentary behavior, as indicated by television viewing time, in childhood and adolescence increases the risk for metabolic syndrome in mid-adult life using data from the Dunedin study. We further extended follow-up of the relationship between childhood and adolescent television viewing and adult obesity and cardiorespiratory fitness in this cohort[9] to age 45 years.

SUBJECTS AND METHODS

Participants

The Dunedin study is an investigation of health and behavior in a population-based cohort. Full details of the study are published elsewhere.[23] Participants were born in 1972 and 1973 in Dunedin, New Zealand. Those still living in the Otago region were invited to the first follow-up at 3 years, when 1037 children (91% of those eligible: 52% male) attended constituting the base sample of the study. Participants have been followed up at frequent intervals throughout childhood and adulthood and were most recently assessed at age 45, when 938 (94%) of 997 surviving cohort members participated. The sample includes the full range of socioeconomic status and is mostly of New Zealand-European ethnicity. Written informed consent was obtained for each assessment, which was approved by the relevant ethics committee at the time (currently the Health and Disability Ethics Committee [17/STH/25/AM05]).

Assessments

At ages 5 (n = 991), 7 (n = 954), 9 (n = 955), and 11 (n = 925) years, parents were asked how much time the participants spent watching weekday television. Participants themselves were asked about television viewing time at ages 13 (n = 850), 15 (n = 976), and 32 (n = 969) years of age. A composite variable of childhood and adolescent television viewing comprises the mean viewing hours per weekday between the ages of 5 and 15 years, as previously reported.[8] Weekday television viewing at age 32 was used as the adult variable.[9] Childhood socioeconomic status was based on the education level and income associated with the highest parental occupation (6 = unskilled laborer, 1 = professional).[24,25] These scores were averaged over the assessments between birth and age 15. Height and weight in light clothing without shoes were measured for 893 participants at age 5 and used to calculate BMI in kg/m^2. Missing BMI values at age 5 were imputed from the measurements taken at age 3 years for a further 120 participants.[8] Time spent doing physical activity was assessed using the modified Minnesota Leisure Time Physical Activity Questionnaire at age 15 years.[26]

At age 45, height (Seca 264 stadiometer, Hamburg, Germany) and weight (Tanita BC-418MA, Tokyo, Japan) were measured in light clothing without shoes to calculate BMI. Waist circumference was measured twice using a steel tape midway between the iliac crest and the lower ribs. Systolic and diastolic blood pressures (BPs) were measured while the participants were sitting and resting using an automated sphygmomanometer (BpTRU, Coquitlam, Canada). Pressures were measured 5 times, and the mean value was used. Cardiorespiratory fitness was measured using a cycle ergometer (Monark 839E, Varberg, Sweden) through a submaximal exercise test. After a warm-up, exercise intensity was modified to maintain a steady-state heart rate of 130 to 170 beats per minute during 6 minutes of exercise at constant power. Maximum aerobic power ($V'O_2$ max) was calculated from the final heart rate using the modified Åstrand-Rhyming method.[8,27] Non-fasting blood samples were collected ~4 hours after lunch. High-density lipoprotein (HDL) levels and triglycerides were analyzed using a Cobas c702 analyzer (Roche Diagnostics, Mannheim, Germany). Glycated hemoglobin (HbA1c) was measured using a BioRad D-100 analyzer (BioRad Laboratories, Hercules, CA). Metabolic syndrome at age 45 was based on the modified harmonized definition with 2 modifications to allow for non-fasting blood samples: a higher cut-point for triglycerides was used and glycated hemoglobin was used instead of fasting blood glucose.[28] The presence of metabolic syndrome was defined as 3 or more of: glycated hemoglobin ≥5.7%; waist circumference ≥102cm (men) or ≥88cm (women); triglycerides ≥200mg/dL; HDL <40mg/dL (men) or <50mg/dL (women); and BP ≥130/85mmHg (or drug treatment of hypertension).

Statistical Analysis

Descriptive statistics for categorical variables are reported as frequency (%) and for continuous variables as means and standard deviations (SD). Childhood and adolescent television viewing was compared between those with and without complete metabolic syndrome data at age 45 using *t* tests. The prevalence of metabolic syndrome in women and men was compared using a χ^2 test.

Associations between childhood and adolescent television viewing and metabolic syndrome at age 45 were analyzed using logistic regression with metabolic syndrome as the dependent variable. All analyses were adjusted for sex. Additional adjustments were made for childhood socioeconomic status, age 5 BMI, and weekday television viewing at age 32. To investigate whether associations differed by sex, the analyses were repeated with a sex-by-television interaction term, and further analyses were split by sex.

We used linear regression to investigate the associations between childhood television viewing and the individual components of the metabolic syndrome, $V'O_2$ max, and BMI at age 45. These analyses adjusted for sex, and further analyses adjusted for childhood socioeconomic status, age 5 BMI, and television viewing at age 32. Models were checked by visual inspection of histograms of the residuals, scatterplots of residuals versus fitted values, residuals versus predictor (childhood television viewing), and leverage versus residual-square plots. Triglycerides, HDL cholesterol, glycated hemoglobin, and age 45 BMI values had skewed distributions. Log-transformation of these variables to approximate normal distributions improved the distributions of the residuals but made no material difference to the interpretation of the analyses. Hence, only the findings from the analyses using untransformed variables are shown.

To explore whether the association between television viewing and metabolic syndrome was due to displacement of physical activity, a post hoc analysis adjusted the association for physical activity at age 15 years.

Analyses used Stata 17 (StataCorp, College Station, TX).

RESULTS

Metabolic syndrome data were available for 879 participants at age 45 and childhood, and adolescent television viewing estimates were available for 870 of these (Table 1). Participants with missing metabolic syndrome data at age 45 (n = 148, 57% men) tended to have watched slightly less television during childhood and adolescence (mean 2.17 vs 2.36 hours, P = .013). $V'O_2$ max was measured in 849 participants at age 45, of whom 841 have estimates of childhood and adolescent television viewing (Table 1).

Metabolic syndrome was more common in men than women (34% vs 20% respectively). Television viewing between ages 5 and 15 years was associated with metabolic syndrome at age 45 in analyses adjusted for sex and with additional adjustments for childhood BMI, childhood socioeconomic status, and adult television viewing (Table 2, Fig 1). These associations were not statistically significantly different between men and women in any of the models (all sex-interaction P values ≥.19). However, when split by sex, the associations were only statistically significant among women (Table 2). Television viewing hours at age 32 were associated with a higher risk for metabolic syndrome at age 45 years (odds ratio [OR] = 1.15; 95% confidence interval [CI]: 1.02 to 1.30; P = .021, adjusted for sex) but not when adjusted for childhood television viewing (OR = 1.10; 95% CI: 0.96 to 1.25; P = .158).

Television viewing between ages 5 and 15 years was also associated with greater BMI values, lower cardiorespiratory fitness, greater waist circumference, and higher systolic and diastolic BP at age 45. No statistically significant associations were found between television viewing and HbA1c, HDL, or triglyceride concentrations (Table 3). There were no statistically significant sex interactions in these analyses (all P values >.05).

Television viewing time at age 15 years was weakly correlated with less physical activity time (sex-adjusted partial correlation r = -0.11, P = .012). Physical activity time at age 15 was not associated with metabolic syndrome at age 45 (P = .731) and the association between television viewing from

TABLE 1 Television Viewing Times, Metabolic and Cardiorespiratory Fitness Values in Male and Female Participants

	n	Male	*n*	Female	*P*
Predictors[a,b]					
Childhood TV, mean (SD) hrs/d	435	2.42 (0.86)	428	2.30 (0.88)	.045
Adult TV, mean (SD) hrs/d	429	1.83 (1.26)	425	2.00 (1.24)	.039
Age 5 BMI[c], mean (SD) kg/m^2	425	16.0 (1.2)	424	15.8 (1.2)	.003
Metabolic syndrome and components[b]					
Metabolic syndrome, *n* (%)	435	148 (34%)	428	86 (20%)	<.001
HbA1c, mean (SD) mmol/mol	436	5.7 (0.6)	431	5.6 (0.5)	.002
Waist circumference, mean (SD) cm	449	96.8 (12.6)	447	87.4 (14.6)	<.001
Systolic BP, mean (SD) mmHg	450	126 (14)	447	117 (14)	<.001
Diastolic BP, mean (SD) mmHg	450	85 (10)	447	76 (9)	<.001
Triglycerides, mean (SD) mg/dL	438	236 (148)	432	140 (84)	<.001
HDL cholesterol, mean (SD) mg/dL	438	47.5 (12.4)	430	60.6 (17.0)	<.001
Other health outcomes[b]					
V'0_2 max, mean (SD)	426	31.6 (6.0)	415	22.1 (5.4)	<.001
Adult BMI, mean (SD) kg/m2	456	28.4 (4.7)	455	28.3 (6.7)	.759

[a] Only participants with measurement of metabolic syndrome at age 45 viewing are included.
[b] Only participants with estimates of childhood television viewing are included.
[c] Includes imputed measures from age 3.

ages 5 to 15 and metabolic syndrome at 45 persisted after adjustment for physical activity time (OR = 1.24; 95% CI: 1.02 to 1.52; *P* = .032). The association between television viewing at just age 15 and metabolic syndrome at 45 also persisted after adjusting for age 15 physical activity (OR = 1.15; 95% CI: 1.04 to 1.27; *P* = .006).

DISCUSSION

In this long-term follow-up of a general population sample, we found that the time spent watching television during childhood and adolescence was associated with a higher risk of metabolic syndrome in mid-adult life. Childhood and adolescent television viewing was also associated with higher values for BMI and lower cardiorespiratory fitness. These findings support our hypothesis that excessive television viewing in childhood increases the long-term risk of metabolic syndrome and is likely to have adverse consequences on adult health.

Our findings that the association between child and adolescent television viewing and adult metabolic syndrome persisted after adjustment for adult television viewing lends support to the idea of a sensitive period during childhood and adolescence, during which sedentary behaviors, such as television viewing, may have a greater influence on adult health than adult behaviors. This is consistent with an earlier analysis from the Dunedin study that found that childhood and adolescent television viewing was associated with obesity and poor fitness at age 32 years independently of concurrent adult viewing.[9] The findings are also consistent with those of Wennberg et al, who reported an association between television viewing at age 16 and metabolic syndrome during adulthood independently of television viewing at ages 21 and 30 years.[2]

The associations between childhood television viewing and adult metabolic syndrome tended to be stronger and were only statistically significant in women. However, none of the sex-interaction terms were statistically significant, indicating that these apparent differences between men and women could be due to chance. Wennberg et al also find no evidence of statistically significant sex interactions but did not present sex-specific findings.[2]

TABLE 2 Associations Between Childhood and Adolescent TV Viewing and Metabolic Syndrome at Age 45 y

	All[a]			Male			Female		
	n	OR (95% CI)	*P*	*n*	OR (95% CI)	*P*	*n*	OR (95% CI)	*P*
Model 1	863	1.33 (1.11 to 1.58)	.002	435	1.21 (0.96 to 1.52)	.113	428	1.51 (1.15 to 1.98)	.003
Model 2[b]	845	1.30 (1.08 to 1.58)	.006	427	1.26 (0.97 to 1.62)	.078	421	1.39 (1.04 to 1.86)	.028
Model 3[c]	837	1.26 (1.03 to 1.54)	.026	422	1.23 (0.94 to 1.61)	.135	418	1.32 (0.97 to 1.81)	.078

Analyses by logistic regression. ORs associated with each additional hr of mean weekday television viewing between ages 5 and 15:
[a] Analyses of both sexes are adjusted for sex.
[b] Adjusted for childhood BMI and socioeconomic status.
[c] Adjusted for childhood BMI, socioeconomic status, and TV viewing in adulthood.

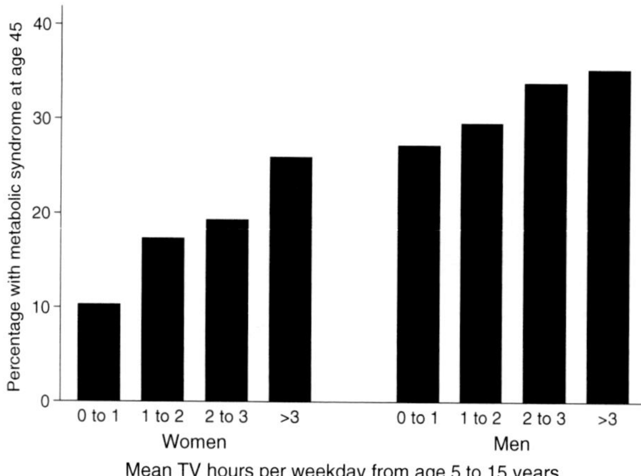

FIGURE 1
Percentage of women and men with metabolic syndrome at 45 years of age according to their reported television viewing time between ages 5 and 15 years.

We did not find statistically significant associations between childhood and adolescent television viewing and HbA1c or triglycerides. This indicates that associations with body weight, poor fitness, and BP may be the primary drivers of the association with metabolic syndrome. This lack of an association between television viewing and HbA1c appears to conflict with the observations that screen time at age 16 predicted adult type 2 diabetes risk in the British Birth Cohort[21] and that television viewing in earlier childhood predicted diabetes risk in the Nurses Health Study II.[20] However, in the British Birth Cohort the increased risk was only present among heavy viewers of 5 hours per day, and few participants in the Dunedin study watched this amount of television. Interestingly, an association between young people's television viewing and adult BP was not observed in an analysis of the Dunedin study at age 26, suggesting that this risk may develop over many years.[8] The clinical importance of this effect, which suggests an approximate mean of a 1.5 mmHg increase in systolic BP for each additional hour of mean screen time, is uncertain, but on a population level, even small changes in mean BP may have major public health implications.[29]

As with any observational study, we cannot prove that the association between childhood and adolescent television viewing and metabolic syndrome at age 45 years is causal. However, there are several biologically plausible mechanisms by which longer television viewing times could lead to poorer long-term health. Television viewing has low energy expenditure and could displace physical activity and reduce sleep quality.[30–32] Our only concurrent estimate of physical activity was at age 15 and a limitation of our analysis is that we cannot fully explore whether the association between television viewing and metabolic syndrome is mediated by the displacement of physical activity. However, although reported physical activity at age 15 was weakly inversely associated with television viewing, it was not associated with adult metabolic syndrome, and the association between television viewing and metabolic syndrome persisted after adjusting for physical activity. This is consistent with previous research suggesting that displacement is not the main mechanism of the longitudinal association between television viewing and BMI or fitness.[8,18,19,33] Screen time may also promote higher energy intake, with children consuming more sugar-sweetened beverages and high-fat dietary products with fewer fruit and vegetables.[32,34–38] These habits may persist into adulthood. However, there is also evidence that longitudinal associations between television viewing and BMI are not due to eating habits.[33]

This study has multiple strengths that support causal inference. It has a high follow-up rate of a general population

TABLE 3 Associations Between Childhood and Adolescent TV Viewing and Adult Health Outcomes

	Model 1[a]			Model 2[b]			Model 3[c]		
	n	Coefficient (95% CI)	*P*	*n*	Coefficient (95% CI)	*P*	*n*	Coefficient (95% CI)	*P*
Components of metabolic syndrome									
HbA1c (mmol/mol)	867	0.30 (−0.15 to 0.76)	.194	849	0.22 (−0.27 to 0.72)	.373	841	0.14 (−0.38 to 0.66)	.597
Waist circumference (cm)	896	2.20 (1.18 to 3.22)	<.001	877	1.58 (0.49 to 2.66)	.004	869	1.22 (0.08 to 2.36)	.036
Systolic BP (mmHg)	897	1.72 (0.65 to 2.78)	.002	878	1.48 (0.35 to 2.62)	.010	870	1.55 (0.35 to 2.74)	.011
Diastolic BP (mmHg)	897	0.94 (0.24 to 1.64)	.009	878	0.74 (−0.01 to 1.50)	.054	870	0.71 (−0.09 to 1.51)	.081
Triglycerides (mmol/L)	870	0.04 (−0.06 to 0.15)	.402	852	0.01 (−0.10 to 0.12)	.842	844	−0.03 (−0.14 to 0.09)	.647
HDL cholesterol (mmol/L)	868	−0.05 (−0.08 to −0.02)	.001	850	−0.04 (−0.07 to −0.01)	.019	376	−0.03 (−0.06 to 0.01)	.133
Other health outcomes									
$V'O_2$ max.	841	−1.01 (−1.45 to −0.56)	<.001	824	−0.82 (−1.29 to −0.34)	.001	819	−0.70 (−1.20 to −0.19)	.007
Adult BMI (kg/m^2)	911	0.98 (0.55 to 1.41)	<.001	892	0.68 (0.23 to 1.13)	.003	887	0.59 (0.11 to 1.06)	.016

Analyses by linear regression. Coefficients represent the unit difference in the outcome associated with each additional hr of mean weekday television viewing between ages 5 and 15:
[a] Adjusted for sex.
[b] Adjusted for sex, childhood BMI, and childhood socioeconomic status.
[c] Adjusted for sex, childhood BMI, childhood socioeconomic status, and adult television viewing.

sample. We were able to control for the potential confounding influence of childhood socioeconomic status. We also adjusted for childhood BMI at the start of documenting television viewing because of the potential for reverse causation: the possibility that some children chose to watch more television because they already have overweight/metabolic problems. We were further able to control for the potential mediating influence of adult television viewing at age 32. We do not, however, have contemporaneous measures of adult viewing at age 45. Other limitations of the study are that television viewing was reported either by the participant or their parent, and we have no way of assessing the accuracy of these reports. However, the use of multiple reports throughout childhood and adolescence is likely to provide a better representation of overall television viewing time than single estimates. Reporting errors in viewing times are unlikely to be biased by the outcome of metabolic syndrome >30 years later, and such errors are more likely to underestimate than overestimate the strength of the association between television viewing and metabolic syndrome. We did not ask about weekend television viewing between ages 5 to 11, but weekday viewing correlates with weekend viewing, and it is unlikely that using weekday averages has substantially affected the validity of our findings.[8] The blood tests were non-fasting but obtained ~4 hours after lunch. We modified the triglyceride cut point to allow for this. We also measured glycated hemoglobin rather than fasting blood glucose. These will have introduced some errors in the definition of metabolic syndrome, but it is unlikely that they will have biased the findings toward an association with television viewing. Participants with missing data for metabolic syndrome at age 45 tended to report watching less television during childhood and adolescence than those with complete data, but it also seems unlikely that these missing data would have substantially altered the observed association between television viewing and metabolic syndrome.

How much screen time should children have? Recent WHO guidelines recommend that children limit the amount of time being sedentary, particularly recreational screen time, but concluded that there was insufficient evidence for a dose-response association and did not specify a time limit.[39] Our data suggest that there is an approximately linear dose-response between young people's television viewing and their later risk of metabolic syndrome (Fig 1). However, our cohort had few screen time options when they were growing up, limiting their exposure. Children today have access to many more screen-based media, greatly increasing the potential for sedentary behavior,[5] and recent data indicate that children have higher screen times.[4,5,40] Although we cannot establish whether these other forms of screen-based activities are associated with long-term health outcomes, such as metabolic syndrome, it seems likely that the consequences would be similar. Our finding that the association between young people's television viewing and the later risk for metabolic syndrome was independent of adult viewing also indicates that there may be a sensitive period during childhood when excessive television viewing has a long-lasting influence on adult health. These findings lend support to the WHO recommendation that children and adolescents should limit their recreational screen time.[39]

This study provides evidence that there is a long-term association between television viewing during childhood and adolescence with metabolic syndrome in mid-adulthood. This adds further evidence of the adverse health effects of television viewing across the life course. Interventions to reduce the time that children and young people spend in screen-based activities may have substantial long-lasting benefits for health.

ACKNOWLEDGMENTS

We thank the Dunedin Study members and their families and friends for their long-term involvement and study founder, Dr Phil A. Silva. We also thank the Dunedin Study Unit Director, Professor Richie Poulton and staff. In addition, we thank Professors Richie Poulton, Terrie Moffitt, and Avshalom Caspi, who collected data used in this report.

ABBREVIATIONS

BP: blood pressure
CI: confidence interval
HbA1c: glycated hemoglobin
HDL: high-density lipoprotein
OR: odds ratio
SD: standard deviation
$V'O_{2max}$: oxygen consumption at maximal exertion

CONFLICT OF INTEREST DISCLOSURES: The authors have indicated they have no potential conflicts of interest relevant to this article to disclose.

COMPANION PAPER: A companion to this article can be found online at www.pediatrics.org/cgi/doi/10.1542/peds.2023-062183.

REFERENCES

1. Viner RM, Cole TJ. Television viewing in early childhood predicts adult body mass index. *J Pediatr.* 2005;147(4):429–435
2. Wennberg P, Gustafsson PE, Howard B, et al. Television viewing over the life course and the metabolic syndrome in mid-adulthood: a longitudinal population-based study. *J Epidemiol Community Health.* 2014;68(10):928–933
3. Wijndaele K, Brage S, Besson H, et al. Television viewing time independently predicts all-cause and cardiovascular mortality: the EPIC Norfolk study. *Int J Epidemiol.* 2011;40(1):150–159
4. Bucksch J, Sigmundova D, Hamrik Z, et al. International trends in adolescent screen-time behaviors from 2002 to 2010. *J Adolescent Health.* 2016;58(4):417–425
5. Bassett DR, John D, Conger SA, et al. Trends in physical activity and sedentary behaviors of United States youth. *J Phys Act Health.* 2015;12(8):1102–1111
6. Ryu S, Kim H, Kang M, et al. Secular trends in sedentary behavior among high school students in the United States, 2003 to 2015. *Am J Health Promot.* 2019;33(8):1174–1181
7. Rideout V, Peebles A, Mann S, Robb MB. *Common Sense Census: Media Use by Tweens and Teens, 2021.* San Francisco, CA: Common Sense; 2022
8. Hancox RJ, Milne BJ, Poulton R. Association between child and adolescent television viewing and adult health: a longitudinal birth cohort study. *Lancet.* 2004;364(9430):257–262
9. Erik Landhuis C, Poulton R, Welch D, Hancox RJ. Programming obesity and poor fitness: the long-term impact of childhood television. *Obesity (Silver Spring).* 2008;16(6):1457–1459
10. Tahir MJ, Willett W, Forman MR. The association of television viewing in childhood with overweight and obesity throughout the life course. *Am J Epidemiol.* 2019;188(2):282–293
11. Engin A. The definition and prevalence of obesity and metabolic syndrome. *Adv Exp Med Biol.* 2017;960:1–17
12. Grøntved A, Hu FB. Television viewing and risk of type 2 diabetes, cardiovascular disease, and all-cause mortality: a meta-analysis. *JAMA.* 2011;305(23):2448–2455
13. O'Neill S, O'Driscoll L. Metabolic syndrome: a closer look at the growing epidemic and its associated pathologies. *Obes Rev.* 2015;16(1):1–12
14. Aguilar-Salinas CA, Viveros-Ruiz T. Recent advances in managing/understanding the metabolic syndrome. *F1000Res.* 2019;8:F1000 Faculty Rev-370
15. Gennuso KP, Gangnon RE, Thraen-Borowski KM, Colbert LH. Dose-response relationships between sedentary behaviour and the metabolic syndrome and its components. *Diabetologia.* 2015;58(3):485–492
16. Wijndaele K, Duvigneaud N, Matton L, et al. Sedentary behaviour, physical activity and a continuous metabolic syndrome risk score in adults. *Eur J Clin Nutr.* 2009;63(3):421–429
17. de Oliveira RG, Guedes DP. Physical activity, sedentary behavior, cardiorespiratory fitness and metabolic syndrome in adolescents: systematic review and meta-analysis of observational evidence. *PLoS One.* 2016;11(12):e0168503-e
18. Grøntved A, Ried-Larsen M, Møller NC, et al. Youth screen-time behaviour is associated with cardiovascular risk in young adulthood: the European Youth Heart Study. *Eur J Prev Cardiol.* 2014;21(1):49–56
19. Sina E, Buck C, Veidebaum T, et al. Media use trajectories and risk of metabolic syndrome in European children and adolescents: the IDEFICS/I.Family cohort. *Int J Behav Nutr Phys Act.* 2021;18(1):134
20. Schmid D, Willett WC, Forman MR, et al. TV viewing during childhood and adult type 2 diabetes mellitus. *Sci Rep.* 2021;11(1):5157
21. Scandiffio JA, Janssen I. Do adolescent sedentary behavior levels predict type 2 diabetes risk in adulthood? *BMC Public Health.* 2021;21(1):969
22. Stamatakis E, Hamer M, Mishra GD. Early adulthood television viewing and cardiometabolic risk profiles in early middle age: results from a population, prospective cohort study. *Diabetologia.* 2012;55(2):311–320
23. Poulton R, Moffitt TE, Silva PA. The Dunedin Multidisciplinary Health and Development Study: overview of the first 40 years, with an eye to the future. *Soc Psychiatry Psychiatr Epidemiol.* 2015;50(5):679–693
24. Elley WB. The Elley-Irving socio-economic index 1981 Census revision. *N Z J Educ Stud.* 1985;20:115–128
25. Poulton R, Caspi A, Milne BJ, et al. Association between children's experience of socioeconomic disadvantage and adult health: a life-course study. *Lancet.* 2002;360(9346):1640–1645
26. Taylor RW, Jones IE, Williams SM, Goulding A. Body fat percentages measured by dual-energy X-ray absorptiometry corresponding to recently recommended body mass index cutoffs for overweight and obesity in children and adolescents aged 3-18 y. *Am J Clin Nutr.* 2002;76(6):1416–1421
27. Cullinane EM, Siconolfi S, Carleton RA, Thompson PD. Modification of the Astrand-Rhyming sub-maximal bicycle test for estimating VO_2max of inactive men and women. *Med Sci Sports Exerc.* 1988;20(3):317–318
28. Alberti KG, Eckel RH, Grundy SM, et al. Harmonizing the metabolic syndrome: a joint interim statement of the International Diabetes Federation Task Force on Epidemiology and Prevention; National Heart, Lung, and Blood Institute; American Heart Association; World Heart Federation; International Atherosclerosis Society; and International Association for the Study of Obesity. *Circulation.* 2009;120(16):1640–1645
29. Cook NR, Cohen J, Hebert PR, et al. Implications of small reductions in diastolic blood pressure for primary prevention. *Arch Intern Med.* 1995;155(7):701–709
30. Sandercock G RH, Ogunleye A, Voss C. Screen time and physical activity in youth: thief of time or lifestyle choice? *J Phys Act Health.* 2012;9(7):977–984
31. Hale L, Guan S. Screen time and sleep among school-aged children and adolescents: a systematic literature review. *Sleep Med Rev.* 2015;21:50–58
32. Kenney EL, Gortmaker SL. United States adolescents' television, computer, videogame, smartphone, and tablet use: associations with sugary drinks, sleep, physical activity, and obesity. *J Pediatr.* 2017;182:144–149

33. Cleland VJ, Patterson K, Breslin M, et al. Longitudinal associations between TV viewing and BMI not explained by the 'mindless eating' or 'physical activity displacement' hypotheses among adults. *BMC Public Health*. 2018;18(1):797

34. Cleland VJ, Schmidt MD, Dwyer T, Venn AJ. Television viewing and abdominal obesity in young adults: is the association mediated by food and beverage consumption during viewing time or reduced leisure-time physical activity? *Am J Clin Nutr*. 2008;87(5):1148–1155

35. Barr-Anderson DJ, Larson NI, Nelson MC, et al. Does television viewing predict dietary intake five years later in high school students and young adults? *Int J Behav Nutr Phys Act*. 2009;6:7

36. Hare-Bruun H, Nielsen BM, Kristensen PL, et al. Television viewing, food preferences, and food habits among children: a prospective epidemiological study. *BMC Public Health*. 2011;11:311

37. Santaliestra-Pasías AM, Mouratidou T, Verbestel V, et al; Healthy Lifestyle in Europe by Nutrition in Adolescence Cross-sectional Study Group. Food consumption and screen-based sedentary behaviors in European adolescents: the HELENA study. *Arch Pediatr Adolesc Med*. 2012;166(11):1010–1020

38. Olafsdottir S, Eiben G, Prell H, et al. Young children's screen habits are associated with consumption of sweetened beverages independently of parental norms. *Int J Public Health*. 2014;59(1):67–75

39. World Health Organization. WHO guidelines on physical activity and sedentary behavior. Report no.: 9789240015138. Available at: https://apps.who.int/iris/handle/10665/336657. Accessed February 26, 2023

40. Twenge JM, Campbell WK. Associations between screen time and lower psychological well-being among children and adolescents: evidence from a population-based study. *Prev Med Rep*. 2018;12:271–283

The Importance of a Life Course Perspective on Media Use

Pooja S. Tandon, MD, MPH

The outsized role of media use in current society is widely acknowledged, as is the need for collective, multifaceted efforts to reduce screen time and mitigate negative consequences for children's health and wellbeing.[1] A significant body of literature reveals the known child health risks of excessive and/or inappropriate screen time, including unhealthy diet, sleep problems, excessive adiposity, poor cardiometabolic health, and increased mental health concerns.[2,3] What is less well-characterized are the long-term consequences of media use in childhood.

In this issue of *Pediatrics*, MacDonell and Hancox use a population-based cohort study from New Zealand with extremely high retention rates (94%, 938 of 997 surviving participants), to demonstrate that television viewing between ages 5 and 15 years was associated with metabolic syndrome, obesity, and poor fitness at age 45.[4] Notably and disappointingly, the findings about the relationship between childhood television viewing and metabolic syndrome at 45 persist after adjusting for television viewing at age 32. Although there is broad recognition of the importance of healthy behaviors in childhood as setting up trajectories of health, there is a tendency to be hopeful that opportunities for course correction exist. Although the benefits of decreasing sedentary behaviors and media use certainly exist in adulthood, as well, these findings underscore the critical and potentially disproportionately larger influence of the childhood years on cardiometabolic health risks. If early media use is, in fact, causally related to adult metabolic syndrome, the mechanism, however elusive, has important public health consequences. Some emerging evidence reveals that the "exposome" early in childhood creates epigenetic changes that predispose to obesity. Seen in this light, limiting screen time in young children takes on even greater urgency.

Interestingly, the association between childhood television viewing and metabolic syndrome persisted after adjusting for physical activity. The authors recognize that this result is consistent with those of other studies, which reveal that the displacement of physical activities by media use in children is not the main mechanism for the negative health outcomes.[5] In fact, in an experimental study that reduced television viewing as a mechanism to reduce BMI, physical activity did not increase although the rate of BMI increase was reduced.[6] Although there is increasing recognition of the interrelatedness of 24-hour movement behaviors (physical activity, sedentary time, and sleep) and their importance for overall child health, there is evidence to suggest that the health consequences of each can be independent of the others. For example, a recent cross-sectional study of US adolescents revealed that a combination of high screen time and low physical activity was associated with overweight/obesity but a high step count may not offset the risk for adolescents with high screen time, and low screen time may not offset risk for those with low step count.[7] However, a few other recent studies do provide an indication that promoting active lifestyles that adhere to healthy 24-hour movement guidelines in terms of adequate physical activity and sleep and limited screen time can be protective in terms of obesity and cardiometabolic risks even into the adult years. Garcia-Hermoso et al

University of Washington and Seattle Children's Research Institute, Seattle, Washington

Dr Tandon drafted the manuscript, approved the final manuscript as submitted, and agreed to be accountable for all aspects of the work.

DOI: https://doi.org/10.1542/peds.2023-062183

Accepted for publication May 8, 2023

Address correspondence to Pooja S. Tandon, MD, MPH, M/S CURE-3, PO Box 5371, Seattle, WA 98145. E-mail: pooja.tandon@seattlechildrens.org

PEDIATRICS (ISSN Numbers: Print, 0031-4005; Online, 1098-4275).

FUNDING: No external funding.

CONFLICT OF INTEREST DISCLOSURES: The author has indicated she has no potential conflicts of interest to disclose.

COMPANION PAPER: A companion to this article can be found online at www.pediatrics.org/cgi/doi/10.1542/peds.2022-060768.

To cite: Tandon PS. The Importance of a Life Course Perspective on Media Use. *Pediatrics.* 2023; 152(2):e2023062183

COMMENTARY

have reported that meeting 24-hour movement guidelines in adolescence was related to a lower risk of abdominal obesity (but not BMI) and type 2 diabetes risk 14 years later in a US cohort.[8,9] In addition, the benefits of engaging in optimal amounts of any of these 3 movement behaviors could have benefits besides weight status and cardiometabolic outcomes and extend into mental health and other domains.

So where does this leave us in terms of prioritizing how and when to intervene with regard to the ubiquitous presence of media in our lives, which is beginning earlier and earlier in childhood? We must first acknowledge that there are some limitations to this study that make the response even more challenging. There have been seismic shifts in media use over the past 40 years, including the advent of the internet, mobile phones, and social media, making it difficult to extrapolate from the sedentary experiences of the cohort participants who were growing up in the 1970s and 80s. Additionally, parent- or child-reported measures of both screen time and physical activity were problematic then, as they are problematic now. Regardless, given that children today are growing up with more screens and fewer physical activity opportunities than previous generations, the findings of this study underscore the urgency of taking a life-course perspective on media use. Obesity and metabolic syndrome are associated with an increased risk of multiple chronic diseases and early death; socioeconomic and racial/ethnic disparities have also been well-documented. Interventions are needed at individual, family, school, community, and policy levels to modify increasingly sedentary and media-infused childhoods while simultaneously studying and advancing strategies to mitigate negative health trajectories to promote population health and health equity. Changing the beginning changes the whole story.

ACKNOWLEDGMENT

Thank you to Dr Dimitri Christakis for his review of this commentary.

REFERENCES

1. Council on Communications and Media. Media use in school-aged children and adolescents. *Pediatrics*. 2016;138(5):e20162592
2. Stiglic N, Viner RM. Effects of screentime on the health and well-being of children and adolescents: a systematic review of reviews. *BMJ Open*. 2019;9(1):e023191
3. Carter B, Rees P, Hale L, et al. Association between portable screen-based media device access or use and sleep outcomes: a systematic review and meta-analysis. *JAMA Pediatr*. 2016;170(12):1202–1208
4. MacDonell N, Hancox RJ. Childhood and adolescent television viewing and metabolic syndrome in mid-adulthood. *Pediatrics*. 2023;152(2):e2022060768
5. O'Brien W, Issartel J, Belton S. Relationship between physical activity, screen time and weight status among young adolescents. *Sports (Basel)*. 2018;6(3):57
6. Robinson TN. Reducing children's television viewing to prevent obesity: a randomized controlled trial. *JAMA*. 1999;282(16):1561–1567
7. Nagata JM, Smith N, Alsamman S, et al. Association of physical activity and screen time with body mass index among US adolescents. *JAMA Netw Open*. 2023;6(2):e2255466
8. García-Hermoso A, Ezzatvar Y, Alonso-Martinez AM, et al. Twenty-four-hour movement guidelines during adolescence and its association with obesity at adulthood: results from a nationally representative study. *Eur J Pediatr*. 2023;182(3):1009–1017
9. García-Hermoso A, López-Gil JF, Ezzatvar Y, et al. Twenty-four-hour movement guidelines during middle adolescence and their association with glucose outcomes and type 2 diabetes mellitus in adulthood. *J Sport Health Sci*. 2023;12(2):167–174

Early Postinjury Screen Time and Concussion Recovery

Molly Cairncross, PhD,[a,b,d] Keith Owen Yeates, PhD,[e,f,g] Ken Tang, PhD,[h] Sheri Madigan, PhD,[e,f,g] Miriam H. Beauchamp, PhD,[i,j] William Craig, MDCM,[k] Quynh Doan, MDCM, PhD,[c,l] Roger Zemek, MD,[m,n] Kristina Kowalski, PhD,[o] Noah D. Silverberg, PhD, on behalf of the Pediatric Emergency Research Canada A-CAP study team,[b,d]

abstract

OBJECTIVES: To determine the association between early screen time (7–10 days postinjury) and postconcussion symptom severity in children and adolescents with concussion, as compared to those with orthopedic injury (OI).

METHODS: This was a planned secondary analysis of a prospective longitudinal cohort study. Participants were 633 children and adolescents with acute concussion and 334 with OI aged 8 to 16, recruited from 5 Canadian pediatric emergency departments. Postconcussion symptoms were measured using the Health and Behavior Inventory at 7 to 10 days, weekly for 3 months, and biweekly from 3 to 6 months postinjury. Screen time was measured by using the Healthy Lifestyle Behavior Questionnaire. Generalized least squares models were fit for 4 Health and Behavior Inventory outcomes (self- and parent-reported cognitive and somatic symptoms), with predictors including screen time, covariates associated with concussion recovery, and 2 3-way interactions (self- and parent-reported screen time with group and time postinjury).

RESULTS: Screen time was a significant but nonlinear moderator of group differences in postconcussion symptom severity for parent-reported somatic (P = .01) and self-reported cognitive symptoms (P = .03). Low and high screen time were both associated with relatively more severe symptoms in the concussion group compared to the OI group during the first 30 days postinjury but not after 30 days. Other risk factors and health behaviors had stronger associations with symptom severity than screen time.

CONCLUSIONS: The association of early screen time with postconcussion symptoms is not linear. Recommending moderation in screen time may be the best approach to clinical management.

[a]Department of Psychology, Simon Fraser University; Burnaby, British Columbia, Canada; [b]Departments of Psychology and [c]Pediatrics, University of British Columbia, Vancouver, British Columbia, Canada; [d]Rehabilitation Research Program, Vancouver Coastal Health Research Institute, Vancouver, Canada; [e]Department of Psychology, [f]Alberta Children's Hospital Research Institute, and [g]Hotchkiss Brain Institute, University of Calgary, Calgary, Alberta, Canada; [h]Independent Consultant, Richmond, British Columbia, Canada; [i]Department of Psychology, University of Montreal, Montreal, Quebec, Canada; [j]Ste-Justine Hospital Research Center, Quebec, Canada; [k]Department of Pediatrics, Faculty of Medicine & Dentistry, University of Alberta, Edmonton, Alberta, Canada; [l]BC Children's Hospital Research Institute, Vancouver, Canada; [m]Department of Pediatrics and Emergency Medicine, University of Ottawa, Ottawa, Ontario, Canada; [n]Children's Hospital of Eastern Ontario Research Institute, Ontario, Canada ; and Independent Consultant, Calgary, Alberta, Canada

Dr Cairncross conceived of the current substudy, wrote the first draft of the manuscript, contributed to the interpretation of statistical analyses, and critically reviewed the manuscript; Dr Yeates conceptualized and designed the larger parent study, conceived of the current substudy, contributed to interpretation of statistical analyses, and critically reviewed the manuscript; Dr Tang conceived of the current substudy, analyzed the data and constructed the figures, and critically reviewed the manuscript; Drs Beauchamp, Craig, Doan, Zemek, and Kowalski conceptualized and designed the larger parent study, contributed to interpretation of statistical analyses, and critically reviewed the manuscript; Drs Silverberg and Madigan conceived of the current substudy, contributed to interpretation of statistical analyses, and

WHAT'S KNOWN ON THIS SUBJECT: The recommendation to restrict screen time after concussion largely reflects expert opinion. In 1 randomized controlled trial, children instructed to abstain from screen time after concussion had a shorter median recovery time than children permitted to engage in screen time.

WHAT THIS STUDY ADDS: Both low and high early screen time predicted more severe symptoms after concussion relative to orthopedic injury during the first 30 days postinjury, but not after 30 days. Other variables had stronger associations with symptom severity than screen time.

To cite: Cairncross M, Yeates KO, Tang K, et al. Early Postinjury Screen Time and Concussion Recovery. *Pediatrics.* 2022;150(5):e2022056835

ARTICLE

Physicians often recommend that children and adolescents limit or avoid use of computers, televisions, phones, and other devices with screens after concussion.[1] Some clinical practice guidelines recommend avoiding screens for 1 to 2 days before gradually resuming use as tolerated,[2] whereas other guidelines mention gradually returning to screen time in the context of return-to-school strategies[3] or imply that screen time restrictions are a component of "cognitive rest."[4] However, advising complete cognitive rest ("cocooning"), including a prohibition on screen time, could conceivably have negative effects on children and adolescents (eg, social isolation, psychological distress).[5–7] The impact of screen time after concussion had not been empirically studied until a recent randomized controlled trial by Macnow et al.[8] Patients aged 12 to 25 years (N = 125) who presented to an emergency department (ED) with concussion were permitted screen time as tolerated or instructed to abstain for the first 48 hours postinjury.[8] Symptom ratings were collected daily for 10 days. The group permitted to use screens as tolerated had a longer median time until recovery (8.0 days [interquartile range: 3.0 to >10.0 days]) than the group instructed to abstain from screen time (3.5 days [interquartile range: 2.0 to >10.0 days]).

Several important questions about screen time after concussion remain unanswered. The long-term effects of screen time on concussion recovery are still unknown. Although screen time within the first 48 hours postinjury could contribute to temporary symptom exacerbation, its longer-term impact has not been examined empirically. The effects of time spent on screens after the first 48 hours postconcussion remain unknown. Whether less screen time facilitates recovery from concussion specifically or benefits the well-being of youth regardless of concussion (eg, decreased sedentary behavior) is unclear. Relatedly, the mechanisms underlying any benefit from screen time restrictions are unknown; however, they may be associated with increased physical activity, which is known to accelerate concussion recovery.[9] The design of the Macnow et al study (ie, 2-arm clinical trial)[8] provides little insight into the association of concussion recovery with the full naturalistic range of screen time. Finally, understanding the importance of screen time relative to other known predictors of recovery, such as preinjury symptoms and early physical activity, would help contextualize clinical recommendations.[10–13]

Our current observational study addresses these questions by exploring the full naturalistic range of screen time over the first 7 to 10 days postinjury and its association with postconcussion symptoms over the following 6 months, while controlling for other predictors of screen time (ie, propensity for higher screen time) and symptom recovery. Furthermore, we compare the association of screen time with symptom recovery in children and adolescents with concussion to those with orthopedic injury (OI) to determine whether screen time is uniquely detrimental after concussion. The OI group controls for factors other than brain injury that can contribute to postconcussion symptom severity, such as pain and posttraumatic stress. We predicted an interaction between injury type (ie, concussion versus OI) and screen time, such that higher levels of early screen time would predict greater postconcussion symptom severity over time in those with concussion relative to those with OI.

METHODS

Design and Setting

This study was a planned secondary data analysis of the Advancing Concussion Assessment in Pediatrics (A-CAP) study,[14] a prospective longitudinal cohort study of children and adolescents who sustained a concussion or OI. Participants were recruited from 5 EDs within the Pediatric Emergency Research Canada network from September 2016 to December 2018.

Participants

Participants ages 8 to 16 years old who presented to the ED within 48 hours of sustaining a concussion or OI were screened for eligibility. Children and adolescents with concussion were eligible to participate if they had experienced blunt head trauma resulting in 1 or more of the following criteria generally consistent with the World Health Organization definition of mild traumatic brain injury (TBI): observed loss of consciousness, a Glasgow Coma Scale score of 13 to 14, or 1 or more acute signs or symptoms of concussion (eg, confusion, headache). Children and adolescents with OI were eligible if they sustained upper or lower extremity fractures, sprains, or strains because of physical trauma, and had an Abbreviated Injury Scale[15] score of 4 or less.

Exclusion criteria specific to the concussion group included neurologic deterioration, neurosurgical intervention, loss of consciousness >30 minutes or posttraumatic amnesia > 24 hours, and bodily injuries with an Abbreviated Injury Scale score >4. Exclusion criteria for the OI group included head trauma, acute signs and symptoms of concussion, or injury requiring surgical intervention or procedural sedation. Additional exclusion criteria for both groups included hypoxia, hypotension or shock; non-English speaking; previous TBI requiring overnight hospitalization; concussion within the past 3 months; history of severe neurologic or neurodevelopmental disorder; psychiatric hospitalization in the previous year; administration of sedative medicine before ED data collection; alcohol or drug use at time of injury; and legal guardian not present.

Procedures

The A-CAP study protocol was published previously.[14] In brief, research personnel collected demographic information, injury details, and acute signs or symptoms of concussion in the ED from medical records and medical personnel using a standardized case report form. Follow-up assessments were targeted for 7 days, 3 months, and 6 months postinjury. At each follow-up, participants and their parents each completed questionnaires regarding symptoms and health behaviors. At the first follow-up, parents also completed measures of preinjury symptoms and health behaviors. In addition, participants and their parents completed remote ratings of postconcussion symptoms weekly during the first 3 months and biweekly from 3 to 6 months postinjury. All participants provided written informed consent or assent. The study was approved by each participating institution's ethics review board.

Measures

The Health and Behavior Inventory (HBI),[16] which is recommended as a primary outcome measure in the National Insitute of Neurological Disorders and Stroke Common Data Elements for sport-related concussion,[17] was used as the primary outcome. The self- and parent-proxy versions provide 2 separate scales for cognitive and somatic symptoms, with higher scores reflecting a higher frequency of symptoms.

The Healthy Lifestyle Behaviors Questionnaire (HLBQ) assessed parent-proxy and self-reported pre- and postinjury engagement in health behaviors, including physical activity and rest, cognitive activity and rest, diet, sleep, and screen time. The scale measuring screen time was used as the primary predictor. Each participant and parent rated the frequency and duration that the child or adolescent engaged in screen time over the previous 7 days. A 5:2 weighted average for weekdays and weekends was computed to provide an estimated weekly average.[18] The total weighted average was used in analyses. Supplemental Information provides information on the development and validation of the HLBQ (see Supplemental Document 1).

Statistical Analyses

Descriptive statistics summarized baseline characteristics. To examine the association between screen time and postconcussion symptoms over time, we fit 4 generalized least squares models, 1 for each of the 4 HBI outcome measures: self-reported somatic and cognitive symptoms and parent-reported cognitive and somatic symptoms. We included both self- and parent-reported screen time as predictors, for 3 reasons: (1) the scale that more accurately reflects a participant's actual screen time is unclear, (2) self- and parent-reported screen time correlated only moderately (Spearman's $r = .60$) in our sample, and (3) we evaluated their combined predictive contribution (ie, joint effect) to postconcussion symptoms. Generalized least squares were applied with a continuous first-order autoregressive[19] structure, with nesting of patients within sites, allowing for correlated residuals from repeated measurement of symptoms and to account for potential clustering because of multisite recruitment. A common set of 27 covariates previously shown to be associated with concussion outcomes[10–12] and parent ratings of preinjury screen time and child and parent ratings of other preinjury and postacute lifestyle behaviors (eg, sleep, physical activity) were included in all models to help isolate the effect of postinjury screen time and reduce potential confounding between the risk for poor recovery and screen time use (eg, children with lower risk for prolonged recovery returning to screen time more quickly) (see Supplemental Document 2, Supplemental Table 3).

To allow for nonlinearity, restricted cubic splines[20] were applied to selected continuous variables considering allowable degrees-of-freedom to maintain an approximate 10:1 observation-to-parameter ratio. For self- and parent-reported screen time and preinjury HBI somatic and cognitive symptoms, 4 knots (ie, pivot points) at strategically-spaced quantiles (0.05, 0.35, 0.65, 0.95) were afforded. For age, social deprivation index, material deprivation index, and preinjury parent ratings of HBI somatic and cognitive symptoms, 3 knots were afforded (0.10, 0.5, 0.90). Linearity was assumed for all HLBQ covariates.

For all models, the initial specification featured 2 sets of 3-way interactions inclusive of both linear and nonlinear components of a continuous predictor's effect. The first set of interactions involved self-reported screen time, group, and time, and the other consisted of parent-reported screen time, group, and time. To simplify the models, we applied a stepwise backward elimination procedure to sequentially remove factors with the largest *P* value until only $P < .05$ remained (on the basis of a multiple degrees-of-freedom Wald χ^2 test, if applicable). As the predictors of primary interest, the main effects of self- and parent-reported screen time were exempted from elimination. Listwise deletion was applied for all models.

To assess the effect of individual predictors and covariates for each model, we report: (1) the Wald χ^2 and associated *P* value, (2) Wald χ^2 minus degrees-of-freedom for evaluating the relative contribution among predictors, and (3) partial effect plots to illustrate the estimated covariate-adjusted relationship between our main predictors of interest and HBI outcomes. Analyses were performed by using *R* version 4.0.3 (*rms* package).[20,21]

RESULTS

A total of 967 children and adolescents (58.1% male) were recruited. See Figure 1 for a participant flow diagram. 829 participants completed the postacute assessment. Of those 829, 117 (14%) participants had incomplete covariate data; therefore, 712 participants were included in all 4 final models. Baseline characteristics are summarized in Table 1. There were no significant differences between those who were included or excluded in the final models in age, sex, other demographics, or preinjury history (see Supplemental Document 2, Supplemental Table 4).

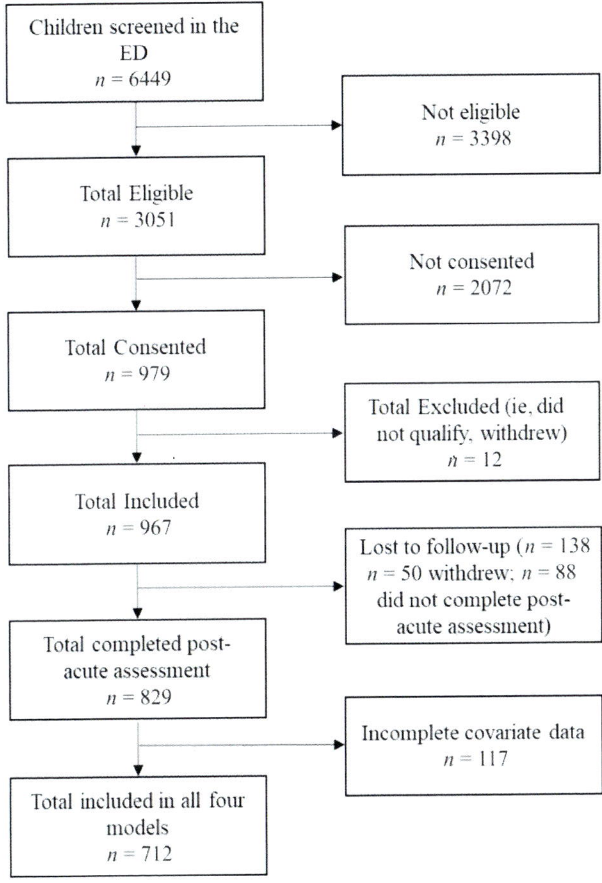

FIGURE 1
Participant flow diagram.

Effect of Screen Time by Group on Postconcussion Symptoms

Our hypothesis that more early screen time would predict greater symptom severity over time in children and adolescents with concussion relative to those with OI was only partially supported. The interaction between screen time and group was not significant for parent-reported cognitive symptoms or self-reported somatic symptoms (see Table 2). In other words, the association of screen use during the postacute recovery period with these outcomes did not differ by group (see Fig 3). The interaction between self-reported screen time and group was significant for self-reported cognitive symptoms ($P = .03$) and parent-reported somatic symptoms ($P = .01$; see Table 2); however, the relationship between screen time and group differences in postconcussion symptoms was not linear. Contrary to our hypothesis, group differences in symptom severity (concussion > OI) were larger at the 25th and 50th quantiles of screen time than at the 75th quantile (see Fig 3). Thus, higher screen time was not uniformly associated with more symptoms in the concussion group relative to the OI group, although group differences were also larger at the highest levels of screen time (eg, 90th quantile).

In all models, symptom severity was higher in the concussion group than in the OI group while holding all other covariates constant over the first 30 days post injury (See Fig 3). Group differences were negligible after 30

TABLE 1 Demographic and Clinical Characteristics of the Total Study Sample

	N	Concussion	*N*	Orthopedic Injury
Age, median (IQR)	633	12.0 (10.2–14.4)	334	12.5 (10.9–14.3)
Sex, *n* (%)	633		334	
Male		379 (59.9)		183 (54.8)
Female		254 (40.1)		151 (45.2)
Familial information				
Parental education, *n* (%)	549		275	
High school or less		86 (15.7)		43 (15.6)
Trades or 2-y college		164 (29.9)		83 (30.2)
Bachelor's degree		206 (37.5)		93 (33.8)
Higher than Bachelor's degree		93 (16.9)		56 (20.4)
Social deprivation index, percentile, median (IQR)	599	41.0 (23.0–66.0)	319	43.0 (23.5–66.5)
Maternal deprivation index, percentile, median (IQR)	599	28.0 (11.0–54.5)	319	27.0 (12.0–56.0)
Preinjury history, *n* (%)				
History of migraine	616	34 (5.5)	329	23 (7.0)
Previous concussion symptom and duration	620		327	
No previous concussion		421 (67.9)		237 (72.5)
<1 wk symptom duration		121 (19.5)		54 (16.5)
1+ week symptom duration		78 (12.6)		36 (11.0)
Retrospective preinjury HBI somatic symptoms, median (IQR)	555	2.0 (0.0–4.0)	281	1.0 (0.0–3.0)
Retrospective preinjury HBI cognitive symptoms, median (IQR)	555	8.0 (2.0–15.0)	281	6.0 (0.0–12.0)
Screen time,[a] mean (SD)				
Preinjury parent	553	5.4 (2.9)	281	5.9 (3.2)
Postacute parent	541	3.9 (3.1)	272	6.0 (3.1)
Postacute self	521	4.7 (3.8)	274	6.1 (3.8)

IQR, interquartile range.

[a] Weighted 5:2 for weekdays and weekends.

days postinjury regardless of screen time (See Fig 3).

Effect of Screen Time on Postconcussion Symptoms Within the Concussion Group

Visual inspection of the relationship between screen time and symptom severity within the concussion group reveals subtle U-shaped distributions in 3 of the 4 models (ie, self-reported somatic, self-reported cogntive, and parent-reported somatic; See Fig 3). Specifically, children and adolescents with concussion who reported the lowest (<25th quantile) and highest screen time (>90th quantile) during the first 7 to 10 days postinjury reported more cognitive and somatic symptoms than those in the25th to 75th quantile of screen time (See Fig 3). Similarly, parents of children with concussion who reported the lowest or highest levels of early screen time (<25th and >90th quantile)

TABLE 2 Summary of Wald χ^2 for Screen Time (Self-PA, Parent-PA, and Joint Effect) Across the 4 Models

	Outcome											
	HBI Somatic Self			HBI Cognitive Self			HBI Somatic Parent			HBI Cognitive Parent		
Factor	χ^2	d.f.	*p*	χ^2	d.f.	*p*	χ^2	d.f.	*p*	χ^2	d.f.	*p*
Screen time self-PA	34.24	12	<.001	10.51	6	.11	18.20	6	.006	5.23	3	.16
All interactions	20.18	9	.02	8.67	3	.03	10.82	3	.01	—	—	—
Nonlinear	23.11	8	.003	8.99	4	.06	10.10	4	.04	5.21	2	.07
Screen time self-PA: group	—	—	—	8.67	3	.03	10.82	3	.01	—	—	—
Nonlinear	—	—	—	8.38	2	.02	6.57	2	.04	—	—	—
Screen time self-PA: time	20.18	9	.02	—	—	—	—	—	—	—	—	—
Nonlinear	18.46	8	.02	—	—	—	—	—	—	—	—	—
Screen time parent-PA	2.12	3	.55	9.15	3	.03	43.79	12	<.001	9.93	3	.02
All interactions	—	—	—	—	—	—	29.33	9	<.001	—	—	—
Nonlinear	1.88	2	.39	0.73	2	.69	21.22	8	.007	4.71	2	.10
Screen time parent-PA: time	—	—	—	—	—	—	29.33	9	<.001	—	—	—
Nonlinear	—	—	—	—	—	—	24.28	8	.002	—	—	—
Screen time self-PA or parent-PA (JOINT TEST)	34.47	15	.003	19.48	9	.02	57.53	18	<.001	16.47	6	.01

d.f., degrees of freedom; HBI, Health and Behaviour Inventory; PA, postacute; —, not applicable.

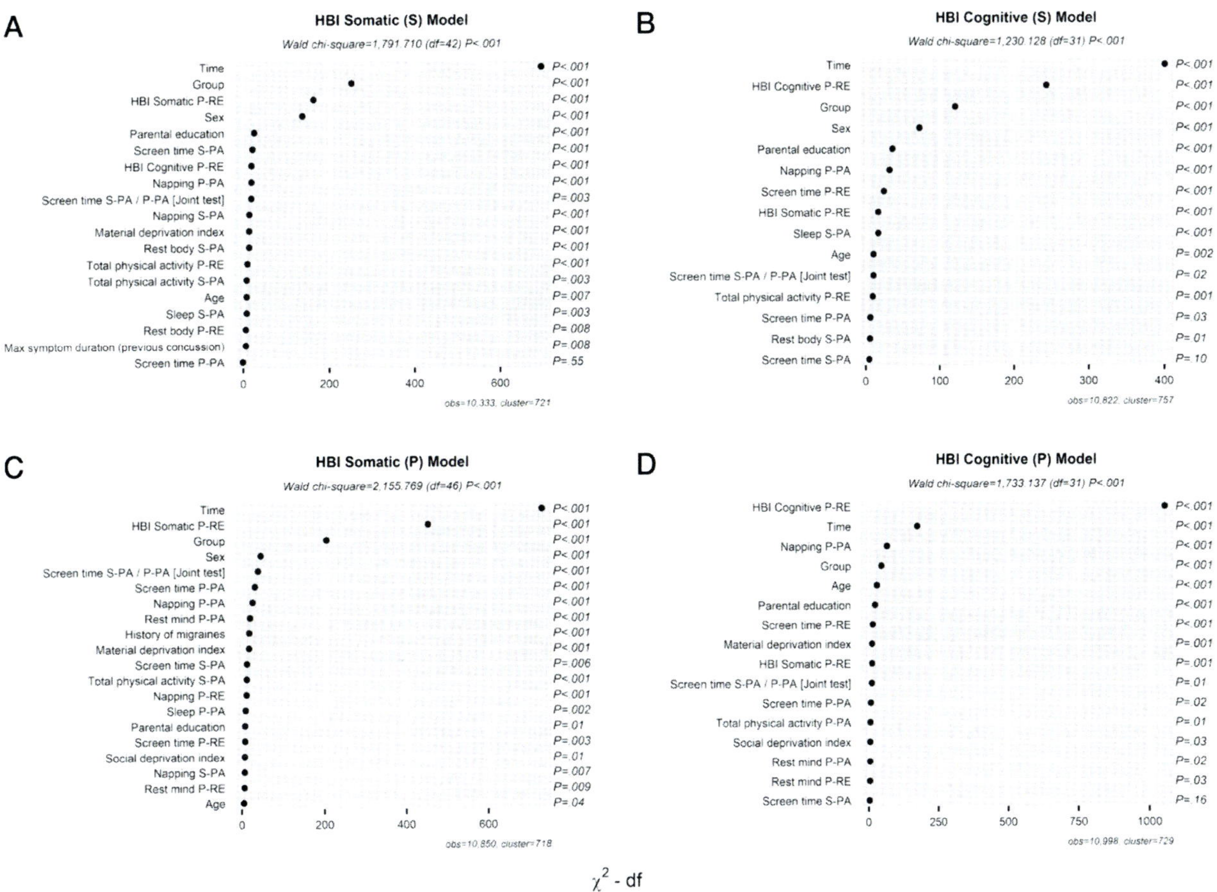

FIGURE 2
Wald χ^2 minus degrees-of-freedom for all (retained) predictors across the models. A, HBI somatic (S) model. B, HBI cognitive (S) model. C, HBI somatic (P) model. D, HBI cognitive (P) model.

reported more somatic symptoms than parents of children and adolescents in the 25th to 75th quantile (See Fig 3). We conducted a supplementary analysis using a validated risk score ("5P")[10] instead of the full set of 27 covariates, to determine if higher risk for developing persistent symptoms moderated the relationship between screen time and concussion recovery. Children and adolescents with concussion with the worst prognosis had similar recovery trajectories regardless of their early screen time (see Supplemental Document 3, Supplemental Fig 6–9).

Effects of Other Preinjury and Postinjury Factors on Postconcussion Symptoms

For all models (see Fig 2A–D), time since injury, group, and preinjury cognitive and somatic symptom severity were more strongly associated with parent- and self-reported symptom severity than self- and parent-reported screen time. Self- and parent-reported screen time accounted for only 0.6% to 3.5% of the proportion of total predictive ability (ie, individual Wald X^2 divided by total Wald X^2) derived from all predictors across the 4 models, compared to 10.3% to 39.6% for time since injury and 2.8% to 14.2% for injury group. Preinjury cognitive symptoms accounted for 60.8% and 19.9% of total predictive ability in models for parent- and self-rated cognitive symptoms. Preinjury somatic symptoms accounted for 21.1% and 9.2% of total predictive ability for parent- and self-rated somatic symptoms.

Several other demographic factors and health behaviors were also important predictors of symptoms regardless of group membership. Female sex predicted higher parent-reported somatic and self-reported somatic and cognitive symptom severity. More postacute napping, more preinjury screen time, and older age also predicted higher self- and

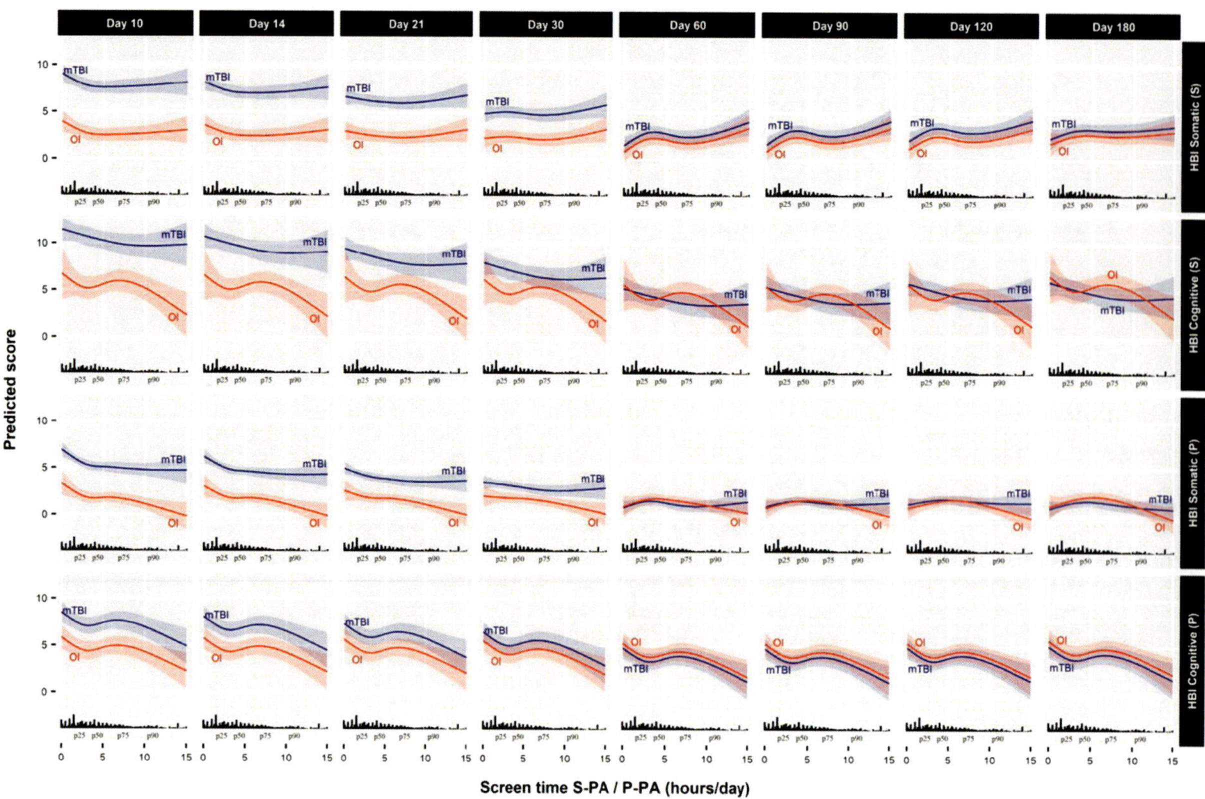

FIGURE 3
Partial effect plots showing screen time effect for concussion across the model.

parent-reported cognitive symptoms, and more self-reported sleep in the postacute recovery period was associated with fewer self-reported cognitive symptoms.

DISCUSSION

This study sought to assess the association between screen time during the first 7 to 10 days postinjury and postconcussion symptom severity over the following 6 months in those with concussion or OI. After controlling for other factors associated with screen time and symptom persistence, greater screen time was not consistently associated with increased postconcussion symptoms. The association between screen time and postconcussion symptoms differed between the concussion and OI groups for only 2 of 4 symptom measures; and for these outcomes, higher screen time was not consistently associated with more symptoms or larger group ifferences (ie, concussion versus OI) in symptoms. Moreover, when present, group differences as a function of screen time were limited to the first 30 days postinjury of the 6-month follow-up period. Although the Macnow et al[5] clinical trial demonstrated that reducing screen time in the first 48 hours postinjury may offer short-term benefits, small group differences in our sample after 30-days postinjury suggest that early screen time is not detrimental for long-term recovery in children and adolescents with concussion.

A novel aspect of the current study was the examination of concussion recovery in relationship to the full naturalistic range of screen time. The screen time abstinence group in Macnow et al (2021) spent an average of 45 minutes per day on screens compared to 3.5 hours per day in the unrestricted screen time group, indicating a comparison of less to more screen time, rather than none to some. This comparison, while important, provides little insight into the association of the full naturalistic range of screen time with concussion recovery. In the current study, the association between screen time and symptom severity was not linear. Participants in the concussion group with low screen time (<25th percentile) reported more postconcussion symptoms relative to those in the OI group than did those with moderate screen time (25–75th percentile). This finding has at least

2 possible explanations. First, a child or adolescent with more severe acute symptoms may self-limit their screen time if it is bothersome or their health care provider or parent may be more likely to restrict their screen use. However, we statistically adjusted for acute symptom severity and other risk factors for protracted recovery, making this explanation less likely. Second, screen time is often used to interact with friends and family or for other tasks like school work. Undue restrictions from screen time after concussion could prevent access to social support or disrupt routines and increase emotional distress,[22] worsening symptoms. In healthy young adults, separation from mobile devices (eg, texting, answering phone calls) can lead to increased physiologic arousal[23] and higher self-reported anxiety,[23–25] especially for heavy phone users.[25]

The "goldilocks" effect we observed in our sample, whereby moderate levels of screen time were associated with less pronounced group differences in symptoms compared to low and high screen use, is not unique to children and adolescents with concussion. The association between screen time and well-being is similarly nonlinear in healthy adolescents.[26] In the digital age, too little screen time may limit meaningful social connections or disrupt routines, whereas too much may disrupt sleep or interfere with engagement in other important activities, such as recreation.[26] As is true for the return to physical activity after concussion,[13] moderation in screen time may be a helpful principle in concussion management.

Consistent with previous studies, greater preinjury cognitive and somatic symptoms,[27] adolescent age,[10,12] and female sex[12,28] were associated with more severe postconcussion symptoms over time. These variables had a larger effect on symptom severity than screen time. Other lifestyle behaviors also predicted worse symptoms, including more postacute napping, less sleep, and more preinjury screen time.

LIMITATIONS AND FUTURE DIRECTIONS

Our study has several limitations. We only measured the duration of screen time. We did not assess the timing (eg, concentrated versus dispersed), quality (eg, active versus passive), or nature (eg, watching television versus social connection) of use. These may be important moderators of the association between screen time and postconcussion symptoms. Second, when parent and self-reports of screen time were discrepant, we could not verify which was more accurate. We used the more conservative estimate of screen time when a large discrepancy existed and truncated values when the sum of reported screen time and sleep duration was >24 hours. Only a small proportion of participants met these criteria (9% for self-report and 7.3% for parent-report). Third, because recruitment occurred in EDs, the results may not generalize to children or adolescents who do not seek care or seek alternative care after injury. We also do not have detailed data on the timing of follow-up care, which could impact recovery. Fourth, children and adolescents who enrolled in the current study may differ from those who did not enroll leading to selection bias. Finally, future work is needed to understand if certain individuals, such as those with vestibulocular dysfunction, are more sensitive to screen use postconcussion.

CONCLUSIONS

High screen time in the first 7 to 10 days postinjury was not strongly associated with worse symptoms after concussion, especially after the first 30 days postinjury, and low screen time was also associated with relatively more postconcussion symptoms. Moreover, other pre- and postinjury risk factors were more important than screen time in predicting postconcussion symptoms. These findings support advising moderation rather than blanket restrictions in screen time, especially beyond the first 48 hours, for children and adolescents postconcussion.

ABBREVIATIONS

A-CAP: Advancing Concussion Assessment in Pediatrics
ASHS: Adolescent Sleep Hygiene Scale
CRSP: Children's Report of Sleep Patterns
ED: emergency department
HBI: Health and Behavior Inventory
HBSC: Healthy Behaviors in School-aged Children
HLBQ: Healthy Lifestyle Behaviours Questionnaire
OI: orthopedic injury
TBI: traumatic brain injury

critically reviewed the manuscript; and all authors approved the final manuscript as submitted and agree to be accountable for all aspects of the work.

DOI: https://doi.org/10.1542/peds.2022-056835

Accepted for publication Aug 16, 2022

Address correspondence to Dr Noah Silverberg, PhD, Department of Psychology, University of British Columbia, 3505- 2136 West Mall, Vancouver, British Columbia, Canada, V6T 1Z4. E-mail: noah.silverberg@ubc.ca

PEDIATRICS (ISSN Numbers: Print, 0031-4005; Online, 1098-4275).

FUNDING: Canadian Institutes of Health Research grant (FDN143304). Dr Yeates was supported by a Ronald and irene Ward Chair in Pediatric Brain Injury from the Alberta Children's Hospital Foundation.

CONFLICT OF INTEREST DISCLOSURES: Dr Yeates is an author of the Health and Behavior Inventory but derives no income from the use of the scale, which is publicly available for free. Dr Zemek is the cofounder, Scientific Director, and a minority shareholder in 360 Concussion Care, an interdisciplinary concussion clinic. The remaining authors have no conflicts of interest to report.

REFERENCES

1. Zemek R, Eady K, Moreau K, et al. Canadian pediatric emergency physician knowledge of concussion diagnosis and initial management. *CJEM*. 2015;17(2):115–122
2. Reed N, Zemek R, Dawson J, et al. *Living Guideline for Diagnosing and Managing Pediatric Concussion*. Available at: https://pedsconcussion.com/. Accessed January 6, 2021
3. McCrory P, Meeuwisse W, Dvořák J, et al. Consensus statement on concussion in sport-the 5th international conference on concussion in sport held in Berlin, October 2016. *Br J Sports Med*. 2017;51(11):838–847
4. Lumba-Brown A, Yeates KO, Sarmiento K, et al. Centers for Disease Control and Prevention Guideline on the diagnosis and management of mild traumatic brain injury among children. *JAMA Pediatr*. 2018;172(11):e182853
5. Halstead ME, Eagan Brown B, McAvoy K. Cognitive rest following concussions: rethinking 'cognitive rest'. *Br J Sports Med*. 2017;51(3):147
6. Silverberg ND, Iverson GL. Is rest after concussion "the best medicine?": recommendations for activity resumption following concussion in athletes, civilians, and military service members. *J Head Trauma Rehabil*. 2013;28(4):250–259
7. Difazio M, Silverberg ND, Kirkwood MW, Bernier R, Iverson GL. Prolonged activity restriction after concussion: are we worsening outcomes? *Clin Pediatr (Phila)*. 2016;55(5):443–451
8. Macnow T, Curran T, Tolliday C, et al. Effect of screen time on recovery from concussion: a randomized clinical trial. *JAMA Pediatr*. 2021;175(11):1124–1131
9. Leddy JJ, Master CL, Mannix R, et al. Early targeted heart rate aerobic exercise versus placebo stretching for sport-related concussion in adolescents: a randomised controlled trial. *Lancet Child Adolesc Health*. 2021;5(11):792–799
10. Zemek R, Barrowman N, Freedman SB, et al; Pediatric Emergency Research Canada (PERC) Concussion Team. Clinical risk score for persistent postconcussion symptomsamong children with acute concussion in the ED. *JAMA*. 2016;315(10):1014–1025
11. Zemek RL, Farion KJ, Sampson M, McGahern C. Prognosticators of persistent symptoms following pediatric concussion: a systematic review. *JAMA Pediatr*. 2013;167(3):259–265
12. Iverson GL, Gardner AJ, Terry DP, et al. Predictors of clinical recovery from concussion: a systematic review. *Br J Sports Med*. 2017;51(12):941–948
13. Grool AM, Aglipay M, Momoli F, et al; Pediatric Emergency Research Canada (PERC) Concussion Team. Association between early participation in physical activity following acute concussion and persistent postconcussive symptoms in children and adolescents. *JAMA*. 2016;316(23):2504–2514
14. Yeates KO, Beauchamp M, Craig W, et al; Pediatric Emergency Research Canada (PERC). Advancing Concussion Assessment in Pediatrics (A-CAP): a prospective, concurrent cohort, longitudinal study of mild traumatic brain injury in children: protocol study. *BMJ Open*. 2017;7(7):e017012
15. American Association for Automative Medicine. *The Abbreviated Injury Scale (AIS) - 1990 Revision*. Des Plaines: American Association for Automative Medicine; 1990
16. Ayr LK, Yeates KO, Taylor HG, Browne M. Dimensions of postconcussive symptoms in children with mild traumatic brain injuries. *J Int Neuropsychol Soc*. 2009;15(1):19–30
17. Broglio SP, Kontos AP, Levin H, et al. National Institute of Neurological Disorders and Stroke and Department of Defense sport-related concussion common data elements version 1.0 Recommendations. *J Neurotrauma*. 2018;35(23):2776–2783
18. Tremblay MS, Carson V, Chaput JP, et al. Canadian 24-hour movement guidelines for children and youth: an integration of physical activity, sedentary behaviour, and sleep. *Appl Physiol Nutr Metab*. 2016;41(6 Suppl 3):S311–S327
19. Pinheiro J, Bates D. *Mixed Effects Models in S and S-Plus*. New York, NY: Springer-Verlag; 2000
20. Harrell FE. *Regression Modeling Strategies*. Cham: Springer; 2015
21. Team RCR. A language and environment for statistical computing. Available at: https://www.r-project.org/. Accessed May 01, 2021
22. Stein CJ, MacDougall R, Quatman-Yates CC, et al. Young athletes' concerns about sport-related concussion: the patient's perspective. *Clin J Sport Med*. 2016;26(5):386–390
23. Clayton RB, Leshner G, Almond A. The extended iSelf: The impact of iPhone separation on cognition, emotion, and physiology. *J Comput Commun*. 2015;20(2):119–135
24. Hartanto A, Yand H. Is the smartphone a smart choice? The effect of smartphone

separation on executive functions computers in human behavior separation on executive functions. *Comput Human Behav.* 2016;64:329–336

25. Cheever NA, Rosen LD, Carrier LM, Chavez A. Out of sight is not out of mind: The impact of restricting wireless mobile device use on anxiety levels among low, moderate and high users. *Comput Human Behav.* 2014;37:290–297

26. Przybylski AK, Weinstein N. A arge-scale test of the goldilocks hypothesis. *Psychol Sci.* 2017;28(2):204–215

27. Ledoux AA, Tang K, Gagnon I, et al. Association between preinjury symptoms and postconcussion symptoms at 4 weeks in youth. *J Head Trauma Rehabil.* 2022;37(2): E90–E101

28. Silverberg ND, Gardner AJ, Brubacher JR, Panenka WJ, Li JJ, Iverson GL. Systematic review of multivariable prognostic models for mild traumatic brain injury. *J Neurotrauma.* 2015;32(8): 517–526

Interventions to Promote Physical Activity and Healthy Digital Media Use in Children and Adolescents: A Systematic Review

Christina Oh, MSc,[a] Bianca Carducci, MSc, PhD,[a,b] Tyler Vaivada, MSc,[a] Zulfiqar A. Bhutta, PhD, MBBS, FRCPCH, FAAP[a,b,c]

abstract

OBJECTIVES: To identify effective interventions that promote healthy screen time use and reduce sedentary behavior in school-aged children and adolescents (SACA) in all settings, over the last 20 years.

METHODS: Searches were conducted from 2000 until March 2021 using PubMed, Embase, Medline, PsycINFO, Ovid SP, The Cochrane Library, Cochrane Central Register of Controlled Trials, Cochrane Methodology Register, and the WHO regional databases, including Google Scholar and reference lists of relevant articles and reviews. Randomized-controlled trials and quasi-experimental studies assessing interventions to reduce sedentary behaviors and screen time in healthy SACA (aged 5-19.9 years) globally. Data were extracted by 2 reviewers and where possible, pooled with a random-effects model.

RESULTS: The review included 51 studies, of which 23 were included in meta-analyses with 16 418 children and adolescents. Nondigital randomized-controlled trials reported a small, but significant reduction of TV-specific screen time (minutes per day) (mean difference, −12.46; 95% confidence interval, −20.82 to −4.10; moderate quality of evidence) and sedentary behavior (minutes per day) (mean difference, −3.86; 95% confidence interval, −6.30 to −1.41; participants = 8920; studies = 8; $P = .002$; moderate quality of evidence) as compared with control groups. For quasi-experimental studies, nondigital interventions may make little or no difference on screen time (minutes per day) or sedentary behavior (minutes per day), given the high uncertainty of evidence. Most studies were conducted in a high-income country. Generalizability of results to low- and middle- income countries remain limited.

CONCLUSIONS: Public health policies and programs will be necessary to reduce excessive sedentary behavior and screen time, especially in the post-coronavirus disease 2019 reality.

[a]*Centre for Global Child Health, The Hospital for Sick Children (SickKids), Toronto, Ontario, Canada;* [b]*Department of Nutritional Sciences, University of Toronto, Toronto, Ontario, Canada; and* [c]*Division of Women and Child Health, Aga Khan University Hospital, Karachi, Pakistan*

Ms Oh and Dr Carducci conceptualized and designed the study, screened the search results, screened the retrieved papers against the inclusion criteria, appraised the quality of papers, extracted the data, completed the data analysis, and drafted the initial manuscript; Dr Bhutta conceptualized and designed the study; and all authors reviewed, revised, and approved the final manuscript as submitted and agreed to be accountable for all aspects of the work.

The protocol for this review was registered within the International Prospective Register of Systematic Reviews (www.crd.york.ac.uk/prospero/) (identifier CRD42020213361).

DOI: https://doi.org/10.1542/peds.2021-053852I

Accepted for publication Feb 16, 2022

Address correspondence to Zulfiqar A. Bhutta, PhD, MBBS, FRCPCH, FAAP, Centre for Global Child Health, The Hospital for Sick Children (SickKids), 686 Bay St, 11th Floor, Suite 11.9731, Toronto, ON M5G 0A4. E-mail: zulfiqar.bhutta@sickkids.ca

ARTICLE

In recent decades, the rise in child and adolescent overweight and obesity is in part attributed to increases in sedentarism among children and adolescents, especially with increasing global urbanization.[1] Going further, the increasing trend of sedentary behavior is particularly concerning with regards to its effects on cognitive, socio-emotional and physical development in this age group, and its future effects on their health into adulthood.[2] Importantly, the measurement of sedentary time is operationalized as activities producing ≤1.5 metabolic equivalents and has often relied on convenient proxy measures such as self-reported screen time, negating the acknowledgment of other forms of sedentary behaviors such as reading, playtime, passive transport and eating, and objective measures using accelerometry.[3] A large body of evidence suggests that greater time spent in front of screens, such as televisions, computers, mobile devices (ie, smartphones and tablets) with apps and social media, and the Internet is associated with poorer cardiometabolic health, shorter sleep duration, unfavorable measures of adiposity and greater mental health outcomes in school-aged children and adolescents (SACA).[4] Moreover, it is also well-established that the abundant access to programming and online content can negatively impact SACA including exposure to risky lifestyle behaviors (eg, unhealthy food, beverage and alcohol consumption) through marketing and advertising,[5,6] issues of "digital dependency" or screen addiction, as well as, risks of exposure to cyberbullying, age-inappropriate and violent content, or sexual exploitation.[7,8] Because of these concerns, both American and Canadian Pediatric Societies issued a recommendation of no more than 2 hours per day of screen time in SACA.[9,10] Furthermore, as screen use has increased considerably around the globe, especially among SACA, it is often at the expense of physical activity.[8] In fact, in a pooled analysis of 1.6 million adolescents (aged 11-17 years), approximately 81% were insufficiently physically active in 2016 globally.[11] In the same vein, the coronavirus disease 2019 (COVID-19) pandemic and its mitigation responses have perturbed routines and lifestyle activities, particularly with the closure of schools and transition to online learning, which may reinforce physical inactivity, sedentary time, and screen use.[12] With this in mind, the World Health Organization 2020 global guidelines call for children and adolescents to accumulate at least an average of 60 minutes of moderate-to-vigorous physical activity (MVPA) per day, and muscle and bone strengthening activities should each be incorporated at least 3 days per week.[13]

On the contrary, digital technologies can also promote beneficial evidence-based outcomes in this population, when used in a safe, responsible, and healthy manner. For example, traditional and innovative media can promote novel ideas and knowledge, and increase social networking and support, opportunities to access health promotion messages and information, as well as interactive eSports participation.[14,15] Previous systematic reviews have investigated the impact of a variety of interventions (single and multicomponent) on sedentary behavior, screen time and physical activity outcomes, which include classroom-based health promotion curriculum, individual counseling for both parents and children, time budgets or time allowances for screen use, media usage diaries, and automated programs that control screen time usage.[16–23] However, these reviews, although insightful, did not exclusively focus on school-aged children and adolescents, and often pooled data from both normal, and overweight and obese participants. Moreover, a previous scoping review conducted by the present authors of this review highlighted the need to distinguish whether nondigital interventions aimed at reducing sedentary behavior and screen time were more effective with certain types of screen use than others. It was found that previous systematic reviews either focused on just one type of screen use (eg, TV use), or grouped all forms of screen time in one pooled analysis making it difficult to parse out distinct intervention effects.[16–22] Therefore, the authors of this review aim to update the knowledge base and evaluate the effectiveness of nondigital interventions to reduce screen use and sedentary behavior, in school-aged children and adolescents aged 5 to 19.9 years globally.

METHODS

Reporting and Protocol

The protocol for this review was registered within the International Prospective Register of Systematic Reviews (PROSPERO #: CRD42020213361). This review was originally designed to evaluate the effectiveness of both (1) nondigital interventions to reduce screen use and sedentary behavior, and (2) digital-based interventions for universal health promotion in school-aged children and adolescents. One search strategy was used (Supplemental Information), and eligible studies were screened together until the abstraction phase, at which time included studies were abstracted and analyzed separately between studies reporting nondigital interventions and those studies assessing digital-based interventions. Given the large number of studies included, the review authors decided to report the evidence synthesis separately.[24] As guidance, we propose a socio-ecological conceptual framework for digital and nondigital health interventions (Fig 1).

Information Sources and Search Strategy

Searches were conducted using a specified search strategy (Supplemental Information) in the following databases: PubMed, Embase, Medline, PsycINFO, Cumulative Index to Nursing and Allied Health Literature, The Cochrane Library, Cochrane Central Register of Controlled Trials (CENTRAL), Cochrane Methodology Register, and the World Health Organization regional databases. The terms were combined with the Cochrane Medline filter for controlled trials of interventions. There were no limitations on geographical settings, publication language, or duration of intervention follow-up. The final search was completed March 16, 2021. Additional details about the search strategy development and other information sources are included in Vaivada et al.[25]

Screening and Selection Process

Although all screening was conducted by a single reviewer, full-text review and data abstraction were conducted in duplicate. Expanded details of the screening and selection process for this review can be found in Vaivada et al.[25] Specific eligibility criteria were used to screen and select studies for inclusion (Table 1).

Eligible study designs included randomized controlled trials (RCTs), quasi-experimental studies (QES), and nonrandomized trials that already assessed the feasibility of the intervention to evaluate the research question.[26] As such, small pilot or feasibility trials without any follow-up larger trials were excluded. Studies were eligible if published in 2000 or after. Classification of high-income countries (HIC) and low- and middle-income countries (LMIC) was conducted according to the World Bank's 2019 fiscal year country income classification. Studies that included both children and adolescent participants without disaggregating the age groups were included, where the majority of the study's sample age fell within the selected age range, or the average mean age reported was between 5 and 19.9 years.

Interventions were defined as any planned action, program, or policy that was implemented to promote healthy digital media use and to reduce sedentary behaviors, screen use, or screen time (Table 1). Eligible comparisons were no

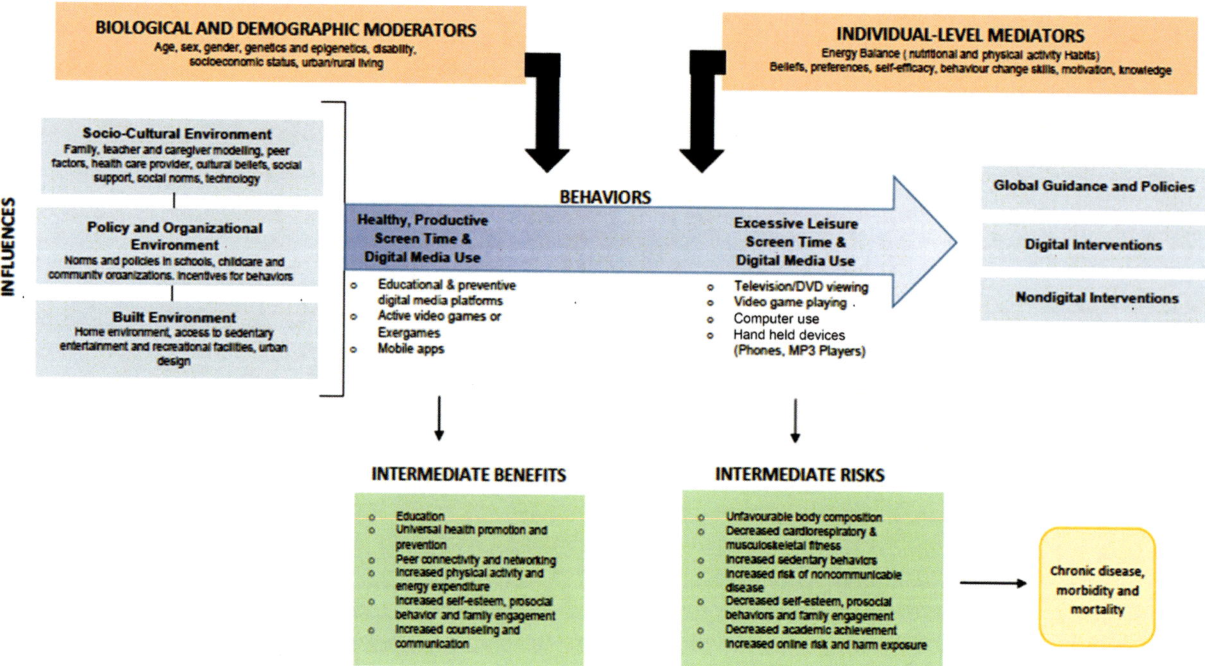

FIGURE 1

Conceptual framework. Child and adolescent screen time and sedentary behaviors are influenced by microenvironments, as well as mediation (individual-level), and moderation (biological/demographics) factors, leading to intermediate benefits or risks, long-term morbidity, and mortality. Such a framework helps illustrate the complexity of these behaviors, guides research, and supports intervention and policy development.

TABLE 1 PICO

	Inclusion	Exclusion
Population	Healthy, male and female children (5–9.9 y) and adolescents (10–19.9 y) with no chronic or existing medical condition, living in a low, middle or high- income country	Unhealthy population, including but not limited to acute or chronic conditions/diseases, genetic diseases Mean age of participants <5 y or >19.9 y
Intervention	Nondigital interventions that aim to reduce screen time and sedentary behavior, with data collected in or after the year 2000 Eligible study designs: Randomized controlled trials (RCTs) Quasi-experimental studies (QES) and nonrandomized trials (NRTs) ■ natural experiment designs ■ controlled before-after ■ regression discontinuity designs ■ interrupted time series	Irrelevant study designs: observational and cross-sectional studies, feasibility studies, reviews
Comparator	No intervention (placebo) Standard arm of care (e.g., existing school programs, activities, or initiatives) Other intervention arms in the case of a multicomponent intervention (e.g., nutrition education arm versus nutrition education + digital component)	
Outcomes	Primary outcomes Screen time or screen use, as author defined (continuous and dichotomous outcomes), including digital dependency, screen addiction or excessive screen use Sedentary behavior Secondary Outcomes Physical activity: all outcomes as author defined pertaining to the measurement of physical activity and energy expenditure	

intervention (placebo), standard arm of care (eg, existing school programs, activities, or initiatives), or other intervention arms in the case of a multicomponent intervention (eg, nutrition education arm versus nutrition education + digital component). Studies were excluded if the primary aim of the intervention(s) was treatment, therapy, and/or management of existing chronic disease (ie, weight loss or treatment of diagnosed overweight and obesity). Only interventions that specifically measured our primary outcomes of interest (screen time and sedentary behavior, as author defined) were included. Although we are aware that physical activity-focused interventions may address sedentary behavior in terms of increases in physical activity or aerobic performance, these metrics were not primary outcomes of interest for this review.

Data Synthesis and Statistical Analysis

Statistical analysis was conducted using Review Manager 5.4 software. Randomized controlled trials and cluster-randomized controlled trials were analyzed separately from quasi-experimental study designs. Meta-analyses were conducted for each outcome of interest, only when there were data fora minimum of 3 studies. Where multiple measures were reported for an outcome in a single study, we used the most commonly reported measure across all included studies. To mitigate heterogeneity within included studies, a random effects meta-analysis was used for all pooled outcomes. Overall effect estimates were considered statistically significant if the associated *P* value was $<.05$.

Because of variation in when studies evaluated outcomes after intervention, when given the choice between after intervention and an alternative, and longer follow-up period, we reported the time point that immediately followed the end of the intervention. This was done where possible across all studies for more consistent and generalizable synthesis. Where possible and appropriate, unit conversions were conducted; this was largely done for screen time and sedentary behavior outcomes where screen time was measured differently (ie, hours/day versus minutes/day). We did not adjust estimates for clustering if cluster-randomized-controlled trials did report adjusted estimates. Sensitivity analyses were not conducted given the lack of studies that could be isolated and provide any meaningful or valuable additional synthesis.

Risk of Bias Assessment

Assessment of risk of bias for included studies were conducted according to criteria and tools outlined in the Cochrane Handbook for Systematic Reviews of Interventions[26] and the Cochrane Effective Practice and Organization of Care guidelines[27] for randomized trials, nonrandomized trials, controlled before-after and interrupted time series. C.O. and B.C. independently assessed risk of bias for each study. These scores were compared and a final score decision was made.

Specifically, randomized trials were assessed using the Cochrane Risk of Bias tool[26,28] across the following domains: randomization process, deviations from the intended interventions (blinding of personnel, participants, and outcome assessment), missing outcome data, outcome measurement, the selection of the reported result, and disclosure of funding and conflicts of interest. Studies were assigned an overall risk of bias judgement accordingly (low risk, high risk, or some concerns).

Quasi-experimental study designs were assessed using the Risk of Bias tool for Nonrandomized Studies of Interventions (ROBINS-I) tool.[26,29] Studies were assessed according to the following domains: bias because of confounding, bias in selection of study participants, bias in classification of interventions, bias because of deviations from intended interventions, bias because of missing data, bias in measurement of outcomes, and bias in selection of the reported result. Each study was assigned an overall risk of bias judgement (low, moderate, serious, and critical risk).

Quality Assessment

A summary of the intervention effect and a measure of quality for all outcomes were produced using the Grading of Recommendations, Assessment, Development and Evaluations (GRADE) approach.[30] The GRADE approach considers 5 domains (study limitations, consistency of effect, imprecision, indirectness, and publication bias) to assess the quality of the body of evidence for each outcome. The evidence was downgraded from "high quality" by one level for serious (or by two levels for very serious) limitations, depending on assessments for risk of bias, indirectness of evidence, serious inconsistency, imprecision of effect estimates, or potential publication bias.

RESULTS

Results of the Search

A database search produced 29 301 records and hand searching revealed another 168 records. After removal of 9132 duplicates, 20 337 records were screened at the title-abstract stage, which identified 680 records for full-text review. Of these, 51 studies (146 articles) met our inclusion criteria for nondigital interventions and 23 were included in the meta-analysis. We excluded 407 records at the full-text review stage for reasons including wrong intervention type, wrong study design, wrong comparator, wrong patient population or wrong outcomes (Supplemental File). Figure 2 shows the study breakdown across exclusion reasons.

Description of Included Studies

Of the 51 included studies, 37 were RCTs,[31–67] 4 were nonrandomized controlled trials,[68–71] and 10 were quasi-experimental studies.[72–81]

Forty-four studies were conducted in HIC, including two studies that were multicenter (Australia, Belgium, Cyprus, Estonia, France, Germany, Greece, Hungary, Ireland, Italy, Netherlands, New Zealand, Norway, Switzerland, Sweden, Spain, United Kingdom, and United States), and 7 in LMIC (Brazil, Ecuador, Lebanon, China, Mexico, and Iran).

Most studies were conducted in school settings, with the exception of 7 studies that were conducted in the community[33,38,49,66,69] or participant's homes.[37,40] Intervention duration ranged from 8 weeks to 4 years. Sixteen studies conducted interventions that ran for 18 months or longer (up to 7 years), whereas another 17 studies implemented interventions that spanned one school year (typically 8-12 months). The remaining studies (n = 17) implemented interventions for a duration of <6 months, and 1 study was unclear in its duration[48] (see Table 2 for characteristics of included studies).

All interventions employed a behavioral modification component including classroom education (ie, didactic, peer-to-peer, or exercise activities), family and community engagement and counseling (ie, newsletters and other media) to promote the benefits of physical activity, the risk of sedentary behavior, and excessive screen use. Some interventions also included other components, such as school and home environment modifications (ie, greater access to healthy foods in the cafeteria, improved physical activity spaces and equipment at school, and implementation of school wellness policies).[32,43,49,51,55,57–60,80] None of the studies disaggregated outcome data based on discrete behavioral and environmental components, providing a limited ability to analyze and understand the specific component effects on outcomes in this age group.

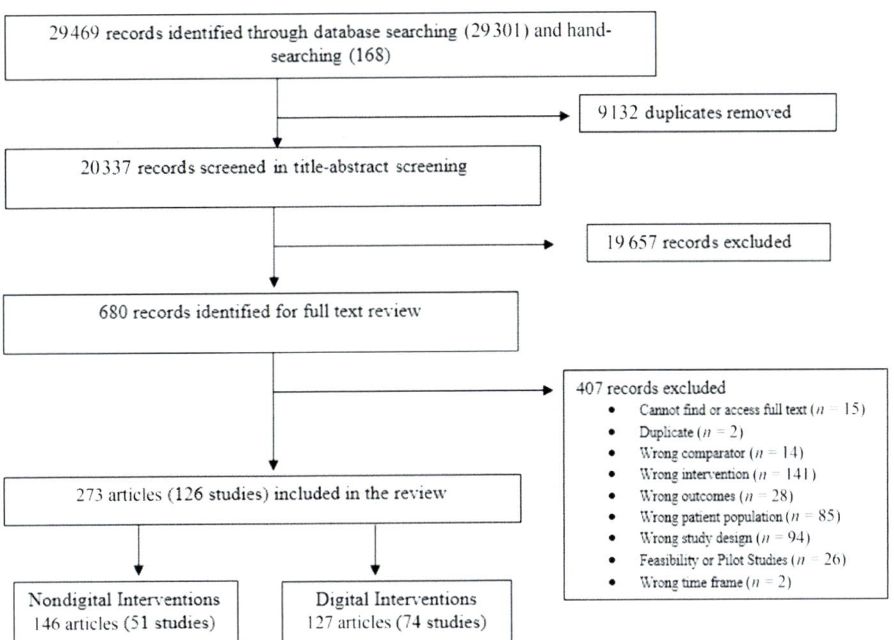

FIGURE 2
PRISMA diagram.

The mean age of participants ranged from 5.0 to 18 years of age. Approximately one-half of the studies (n = 23) reported a mean age <10 years, 11 studies included both school-aged children and adolescents, and the remaining studies reporting mean ages between 11 and 18 years.

Risk of Bias

The majority of nondigital based RCTs (28 of 37) were high risk of bias, six had some concerns,[31,32,43,52,66,67] and three were of low risk.[48,51,53] Randomization was considered adequate in 24 trials. A common reason for downgrading study quality was concerns with risk of bias due to deviations from the intended interventions, involving allocation concealment blinding processes, and outcome assessment. Allocation concealment was unclear in most studies (26 of 37). Blinding of participants and personnel was considered poor or unclear, with only four trials blinding participants,[48,51–53] 9 trials blinding personnel,[31–33,46,48,51–54] and 7 trials blinding outcome assessment.[32,48,51–53,59,67] Other reasons for downgrading study quality included attrition bias, disclosed funding and conflicts of interest. Attrition bias was considered high risk in 6 trials, with loss to follow-up ranging from 22%[44,56] to 32%.[60] The majority of studies disclosed funding, except for three studies,[35,38,47] whereas 9 studies did not declare their conflicts of interest.[34,35,53,55,58,60,62,63,78]

Of the nonrandomized controlled trials and QES, the majority of studies (9 of 14) were judged as having a moderate risk of bias because of poor adjustment of confounding variables, missing outcome data, subjective outcome assessments, and selected reported results. Three studies had an overall low risk of bias,[69,70,76] whereas two studies had serious risk.[74,78]

Effect of the Interventions

Eighteen studies were included in the RCT meta-analyses for nondigital based interventions,[31,32,36–38,40,43,47–53,56,57,60,62,68] whereas 5 studies were included in QES meta-analyses.[68,70,71,73,81]

When compared with control groups, nondigital interventions probably results in a slight reduction of TV-specific screen time (minutes per day) (mean difference [MD], −12.46; 95% confidence interval [CI], −20.82 to −4.10; participants = 6097; studies = 6; I^2 = 59%; P = .004; moderate quality of evidence). Additionally, nondigital interventions may result in a reduction in screen time (all media types) (minutes per day) (MD −11.45; 95% CI, −19.18 to −3.73; participants = 7070; studies = 9; I^2= 38%; P = .004; low quality of evidence) (Figs 3 and 4).

TABLE 2 Characteristics of Included Studies (Nondigital Based Interventions for Screen Time and Sedentary Behaviors)

Source	Country, World Bank Region[a]	Study Design[b]	Participants (Sample Size, Age Range, Description)	Intervention		Reported Outcomes[c]
				Duration, Frequency	Description	
Andrade et al (32)	Ecuador, LAC	cRCT	N =1440, grades 8–9; mean age 12.8 (SD 0.8) y; 62.4% female	2 mo, every 2 wk	Classroom education on physical activity and screen time behavior; school environment modifications and parental workshops (ACTIVITAL)	ST
Aragon Neely et al (33)[d]	USA, NA	RCT	N = 439; 2–12 y; median age 5.0 y	4 mo	Play Nicely video or handout 'Pulling the Plug on TV violence'	ST, PA
Bickham et al (72)[d]	USA, NA	QES	N = 529; grades 6–8 living in rural school district	3-4 mo (1 semester)	Peer-to-peer education about health effects of excessive screen media use (Take the Challenge)	ST, PA
Breslin et al (73)	Ireland, ECA	QES	N = 416; 8–9 y; primary school children from lower socioeconomic backgrounds	12 wk, weekly	Education and activities on effects of physical activity on health and nutrition (Sport for LIFE)	ST, PA, SB
Colin-Ramirez et al (34)[d]	Mexico, LAC	RCT	N = 619; 8–10 y; mean age 9.4 (SD 0.7) primary school students from low SES; ~48% female	1 y, weekly	Education on physical activity and sedentary behavior; exercise breaks and physical activity classes (RESCATE)	ST
Cong et al (74)[d]	USA, NA	QES	N = 416; 5–9 y; Hispanic children from low-income backgrounds	22 mo	Education and exercise activities to reduce TV and video game screen time and increase physical activity (Transformacion Para Salud)	ST
Contento et al (35)[d]	USA, NA	cRCT	N = 1136; inner city seventh grade students; mean age 12 y	8-10 wk	Education on healthy food and activity choices and agency (C3 Intervention)	ST
Cronholm et al (70)	Sweden, ECA	CBA	N = 228; mean age 14.8y; 59% boys	7 y	Increase in physical activity curriculum	ST, PA
Duncan et al (36)	New Zealand, EAP	cRCT	N = 675; primary school students; 7–10 y	1 y	Education to promote physical activity and healthy eating (Healthy Homework)	ST, PA, SB

TABLE 2 Continued

Source	Country, World Bank Region[a]	Study Design[b]	Participants (Sample Size, Age Range, Description)	Intervention: Duration, Frequency	Intervention: Description	Reported Outcomes[c]
Epstein et al (37)	USA, NA	RCT	$N = 70$; 4–7 y; ≥75th BMI percentile for age and sex; participate in at least 14 h of RV viewing and computer game per week	2 y	TV monitoring device recorded number of minutes of use at the home; education on alternatives to sedentary behaviors; tailored monthly newsletter for parents	ST, PA
Escobar-Chaves et al (38)	USA, NA	RCT	$N = 202$; 6–9 y; children from large, urban multiethnic population	6 mo, biweekly	2-h workshop and 6 bimonthly newsletters to reduce screen time/TV use	ST
Filho et al 2019 (39)[d]	Brazil, LAC	cRCT	$N = 1272$; grades 7–9 students from full-time schools in neighborhoods of socially vulnerable areas; 11–18 y	4 mo, weekly	Education on excessive screen time and opportunities for increased physical activity at school; health promotion posters and flyers (Fortaleça sua Saúde)	ST, PA
Foster et al (60)	USA, NA	cRCT	$N = 1349$; grades 4–6 students from schools where 50% of the students are eligible for free or reduced-price meals; mean age 11 y	2 y	Nutrition education; nutrition policy and social marketing at school; parent outreach and involvement (School Nutrition Policy Initiative)	ST, SB
Fulkerson et al (40)	USA, NA	RCT	$N = 160$; 8–12 y with BMI >50th percentile for age	1 y, monthly	Education for student and parent on nutrition and physical activity (HomePlus)	ST
Gentile et al (41)[d]	USA, NA	RCT	$N = 1323$; grades 3–5 students; mean age 9.6 y; 53% female	8 mo	Paid and unpaid advertising and media promotion, and education on limiting screen time use, increasing physical activity, and improving nutrition (Switch what you Do, View, and Chew)	ST, PA
Gholamian et al (75)[d]	Iran, MENA	QES	$N = 120$; adolescent girls with internet addiction from high schools of	2 mo	2-d education session for students; 1 session for parents about	ST

TABLE 2 Continued

Source	Country, World Bank Region[a]	Study Design[b]	Participants (Sample Size, Age Range, Description)	Intervention		Reported Outcomes[c]
				Duration, Frequency	Description	
			same social and economic situation; 16–17 y		excessive internet use and related health effects	
Habib-Mourad et al (42)[d]	Lebanon, MENA	cRCT	N = 2276; grades 4–5; 9–11 y	3 mo, weekly	Education and interactive activities on decreasing sedentary behavior, increasing physical activity, and increasing healthy food consumption (Health-E-PALS)	PA, SB
Harrison et al (76)[d]	Ireland, ECA	QES	N = 312; students from schools in areas of social disadvantage; mean age 10.2 (SD 0.7) y	16 wk, weekly	Education on increasing physical activity and reducing screen time with personal workbooks to record leisure time/screen time use (Switch off -Get Active)	ST, PA
Jones et al (43)	USA, NA	cRCT	N = 718; girls in the sixth grade enrolled in 2 semesters of physical education; mean age 11.6 (SD 0.4)	18 mo	Health curriculum and peer-based behavioral journalism, physical education program and improvement of school food service (IMPACT)	ST, PA, SB
Kipping et al (31)	United Kingdom, ECA	cRCT	N = 2221; grades 4–6; 8–11 y	6-7 mo	Education on nutrition and reduced screen time use with homework activities; newsletters sent to parents (AFLY5)	ST, PA, SB
Knebel et al (44)[d]	Brazil, LAC	cRCT	N = 999; grades 7–9	10 mo	Education on health eating, physical activity, and screen time use; school environment modifications; teacher training (Movimente)	ST
Kobel et al (45)[d]	Germany, ECA	cRCT	N = 1943; grades 1–2; 48.8% female; mean age 7.1 (SD 0.6)	1 y, mixed	Education and alternative recreational activities for physical activity and reduced	ST, PA

TABLE 2 Continued

Source	Country, World Bank Region[a]	Study Design[b]	Participants (Sample Size, Age Range, Description)	Intervention: Duration, Frequency	Intervention: Description	Reported Outcomes[c]
					screen time use (Join the Healthy Boat)	
Lindenberg et al (46)[d]	Germany, ECA	cRCT	N = 2430; students at risk for internet use disorder (CIUS≥20); 12–18 y	1 y	Education focused on internet use disorder and related behaviors and mental health (PROTECT)	ST
Llargues et al (47)	Spain, ECA	cRCT	N = 426; 5–6 y; primary school children	2 y	Education of healthy dietary habits and physical activity	ST, PA
Lloyd et al (48)	United Kingdom, ECA	cRCT	N = 1324; 9–10 y; students from state-run primary and junior schools	Unclear duration, daily	Education on healthy lifestyle behaviors; creation of supportive environments and personal goal setting with parental support (Healthy Lifestyles Program)	PA, SB
Morgan et al (66)[d]	Australia, EAP	RCT	N = 115 fathers (29–53 y) and 153 daughters (4–12 y); mean age 7.7 (SD 1.8)	2 mo	Education on physical activity, socio-emotional wellbeing, and engagement in activities (DADEE program)	ST, PA
Novotny et al (49)	USA, NA	cRCT	N=4333; 2–8 y	2 y	Increased access to healthy foods and environments for safe play; strengthened school wellness policies; social marketing and training (Children's Healthy Living Program)	ST, PA
Neumark-Sztainer et al (61)[d]	USA, NA	cRCT	N = 356 girls; mean age 15.9 (SD 1.2); 75% were racial/ ethnic minorities	9 mo, 2 cohorts, weekly	Physical education, individual counseling, parent outreach and lunch get-togethers (New Moves)	ST, PA, SB
Nyberg et al (50)	Sweden, ECA	cRCT	N = 378; 6-y old students living in disadvantaged areas	6 mo	Education and motivational interviewing on physical activity, reducing screen time and healthy eating (Healthy School Start)	ST, PA, SB

TABLE 2 Continued

Source	Country, World Bank Region[a]	Study Design[b]	Participants (Sample Size, Age Range, Description)	Intervention		Reported Outcomes[c]
				Duration, Frequency	Description	
Pardo et al (77)[d]	Spain, ECA	QES	*N* = 682; 12–15 y	3 y, daily	Education and extracurricular activities on reducing screen time and sweetened beverage consumption, and increasing physical activity (Sigue la Huella (Follow the Footstep))	ST, SB
Puder et al (51)	Switzerland, ECA	cRCT	*N* = 652; predominately migrant children; mean age 5.2 (SD 0.6)	9.5 mo, mixed	Physical activity sessions and environmental changes, parental education, teacher training and healthy food promotion (Ballabeina)	ST, PA
Racine et al (78)[d]	USA, NA	QES	*N* = 1027; 8–13 y; 60% female	12 wk, weekly	Physical activities and education on healthy lifestyle behaviors, nutrition and staying active	ST, PA
Robinson (53)	USA, NA	RCT	*N* = 198; grades 3–4; 8–10 y; mean age 8.9 y	1 y	Education on self-monitoring and self-reporting of screen time use	ST, PA, SB
Robinson et al (52)	USA, NA	RCT	*N* = 284; 8–10 y African American girls from low-income areas; with BMI ≥25th percentile for age and/or at least 1 overweight parent or guardian	2 y	Afterschool dance intervention offered 5 d/wk (Stanford GEMS)	ST, PA
Sahota et al (54)[d]	United Kingdom, ECA	cRCT	*N* = 636 children; 7–11 y; mean age 8.4 y (SD 0.63)	1 y	Active program promoting lifestyle education, modification of school meals, school action plans (APPLES)	PA, SB
Salmon et al (55)[d]	Australia, EAP	cRCT	*N* = 311; grade 5 students from primary schools from low socioeconomic areas; 10.6 y	9 mo	Behavior modification and functional movement intervention, in addition to physical activity classes (Switch-Play)	ST, PA

TABLE 2 Continued

Source	Country, World Bank Region[a]	Study Design[b]	Participants (Sample Size, Age Range, Description)	Intervention: Duration, Frequency	Intervention: Description	Reported Outcomes[c]
Salmon et al (64)[d]	Australia, EAP	cRCT	N = 293 children; 7–9 y, mean age 8.0 (SD 1.3)	18 mo	Education and environmental changes including signage, physical activity equipment (Transform Us!)	ST
Salway et al (65)[d]	United Kingdom, ECA	cRCT	N = 1558 girls, 13–14 y	5 mo	Peer-led intervention to promote physical activity (PLAN-A)	ST, PA, SB
Schmidt et al (71)	Norway, ECA	nRCT	N = 813; 13–15 y	7 mo	Teacher-led activities to promote healthy lifestyles (Active and Healthy Kids Program)	PA, ST
Sevil et al (81)	Spain, ECA	QES	N = 225; 12–14 y; mean age 13.06 ± 0.61; 52.9% girls	One school year	A multicomponent intervention with curricular (ie, tutorial action plan, interdisciplinary project, and school break) and extracurricular (ie, family involvement, institutional and noncurricular activities, and dissemination of health information and events) actions to promote adolescents' healthy lifestyles	ST, PA, SB
Simon et al (62)	France, ECA	RCT	N = 954; 11–12 y; mean age 11.7 (SD 0.6) y	4 y, weekly	Education on physical activity and sedentary behavior; new opportunities for physical activity during school/after-school hours (ICAPS)	ST, PA
Spruijt-Metz et al (63)[d]	USA, NA	cRCT	N = 459; middle school girls; 75% Latina; mean age 12.5 y	5-7 d, daily	Education and activities on physical activity and sedentary behavior (Get Moving!)	ST, PA
Tarro et al (56)	Spain, ECA	cRCT	N = 702; children and adolescents from primary and high schools in disadvantaged	9 mo	Peer-led education and social marketing health-promoting activities to promote physical	ST, PA

TABLE 2 Continued

Source	Country, World Bank Region[a]	Study Design[b]	Participants (Sample Size, Age Range, Description)	Intervention		Reported Outcomes[c]
				Duration, Frequency	Description	
			neighborhoods; 9–11 y		activity, healthy eating and reduce screen time (EYTO-Kids project)	
Van Kann et al (79)[d]	Netherlands, ECA	QES	*N* = 791; grades 6–7; 8–11 y	1 y, daily	School environment modifications including increased recess, new equipment, and opportunities for physical activity (Active Living Project)	PA, SB
Van Lippevelde et al (57)	Germany, Belgium, Greece, Hungry and Norway, ECA	cRCT	*N* = 3325; 10–12 y; mean age 11.2 y	2 mo, weekly	Education on increased awareness about sedentary behaviors; goal setting and home environment modifications (UP4FUN)	ST, SB
Van Nassau et al (68)	Netherlands, ECA	nRCT	*N* = 2088; 12–14 y	20 mo	Education on physical activity and other healthy lifestyle behaviors (DOiT)	ST, PA
van Stralen et al (80)[d]	Netherlands, ECA	QES	*N* = 600; grades 6–7; 8–12 y; mean age 9.8 (SD 0.7 y); 51% girls; 13% Dutch ethnicity; 35% overweight	20 mo	Increased sports participation; personal workbooks for children and parents; parental information about developing supportive home environments (JUMP-in)	ST, PA
Veldman et al (67)[d]	Australia, EAP	cRCT	*N* = 60; 5–10 y; mean age 7.7 SD 1.8, 50% girls	6 mo	Promotion of physical activity through team sport activities and academic enrichment	PA, SB
Verbestel et al (69)[d]	Belgium, Cyprus, Estonia, Germany, Hungary, Italy, Spain, and Sweden, ECA	nRCT	*N* = 9184; 2–9.9 y	2 y	Education on healthy lifestyle behaviors including decreased daily screen time use and increasing daily physical activity (IDEFICS)	PA, SB

TABLE 2 Continued

Source	Country, World Bank Region[a]	Study Design[b]	Participants (Sample Size, Age Range, Description)	Intervention: Duration, Frequency	Intervention: Description	Reported Outcomes[c]
Wang et al (58)[d]	USA, NA	RCT	*N* = 450; grades 5–8 African American adolescents in public schools in low socioeconomic urban areas; 9–14 y	18 mo	School and community environment enrichment and modifications; family support to reduce sedentary behavior and increase other healthy behaviors (HEALTH-KIDS)	PA, ST
Xu et al (59)[d]	China, EAP	cRCT	*N* = 1182; grade 4 students; mean age 10.2 (SD 0.5)	1 y (2 school semesters), mixed	Education on healthy behaviors; school environment promotion; family involvement and fun programs/ events for students (CLICK-Obesity)	ST

[a] World Bank regions: EAP, East Asia Pacific; ECA, Europe & Central Asia; LAC, Latin America & Caribbean; MENA, Middle East & North Africa; NA, North America; SA, South Asia; SSA, Sub-Saharan Africa.

[b] CBA, controlled before-after; cRCT, cluster randomized controlled trial; nRCT, nonrandomized controlled trial; QES, quasi-experimental study; RCT, randomized controlled trial.

[c] PA, physical activity; SB, sedentary behavior; ST, screen time.

[d] Studies were excluded from analysis for reasons including, unclear sample sizes at follow-up or post-intervention, lack of disaggregation of data between intervention and control groups, no outcomes of interest.

However, these interventions may make little to no difference on reducing screen time specific to computer gaming or video gaming (minutes per day) given the high uncertainty of the evidence (MD, −3.51; 95% CI, −9.02 to 2.01; participants = 5365; studies = 5; I^2 = 56%; *P* = .21; very low quality of evidence). With regards to sedentary behavior, nondigital interventions probably result in a slight reduction of sedentary time (minutes per day) as compared with controls (MD, −3.86; 95% CI, −6.30 to −1.41; participants = 8920; studies = 8; I^2 = 0%; *P* = .002; moderate quality of evidence) (Figs 5 and 6).

The effects of nondigital interventions on MVPA (minutes per day) as compared with control groups may make little to no difference on increasing MVPA (MD, −0.07; 95% CI, −1.83 to 1.69; participants = 5540; studies = 6; I^2 = 31%; *P* = .94; low quality of evidence). Two RCTs reported accelerometer data for weekdays and weekends (counts per minute or steps per day).[52,69] However, both studies found nonsignificant differences between intervention and control groups at follow-up, after adjustment (Fig 7).

With regards to QES, nondigital interventions may make little to no difference on reducing screen time of all media types (minutes per day) (MD, −26.76; 95% CI, −67.31 to 13.79; participants = 1984; studies = 3; I^2 = 97%; *P* = .20; very low quality of evidence) or sedentary behavior (minutes per day) (MD, −9.65; 95% CI, −41.05 to 21.75; participants = 1010; studies = 3; I^2 = 90%; *P* = .60; very low quality of evidence), given the high uncertainty of the evidence (Supplemental Information).

DISCUSSION

This review provides a comprehensive appraisal of 51 studies conducted in 24 countries, evaluating nondigital interventions aimed at minimizing screen time and sedentary behavior in healthy children and adolescents of normal BMI. This review analyzed over 16 000 children and adolescents and included 19 new trials, conducted in the last 5 years.[17,31,36,39,40,44–46,]

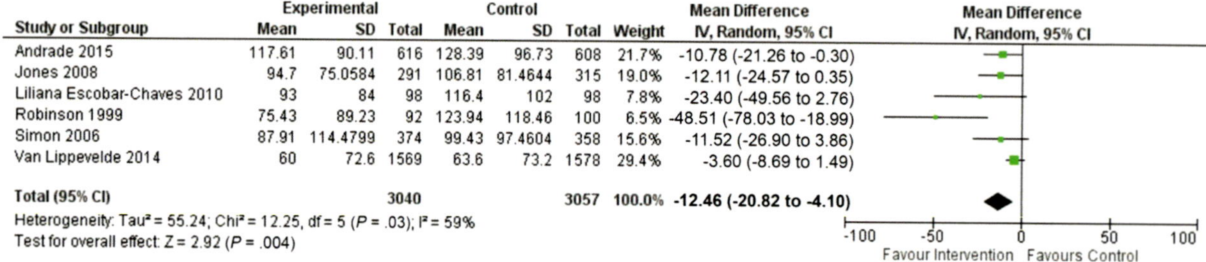

FIGURE 3

Forest plot of screen time (author-defined TV; minutes per day).

48–50,56,65–67,69–71,81 Our review suggests that nondigital interventions indeed resulted in a small, but significant reduction in sedentary behavior. This review also indicates that nondigital interventions were most successful at reducing TV screen time compared with other forms of screen time, such as computer and gaming. Although there are many previous reviews that evaluated both single and multicomponent interventions in a variety of populations, including overweight and obese participants, it was important that this review focus solely on healthy children and adolescents, to provide greater insight into the possible effectiveness and potential of these interventions in public health prevention initiatives.

Previous systematic reviews[16–23] found similar results, whereby screen time from all media types was reduced by 10 to 20 minutes per day in intervention groups when compared with control groups. However, these meta-analyses varied in their inclusion criteria of participants (ie, exclusively overweight and obese populations) and in some cases, both preschool and adult populations. For example, van Grieken et al[19] reported adolescent screen time use was reduced by a mean of −17.95 minutes per day (95% CI, −26.61 to −9.28) in a pooled analysis of 13 studies including overweight and obese adolescents. Likewise, Wahi et al[20] found in a pooled analysis of 9 studies in children (aged 3.9 to 11.7 years), intervention groups reduced screen time by a mean of −0.90 hours per week (95% CI, −3.47 to 1.66), however these results were not significant (P = .49). Albeit in the long-term, this small reduction does equate to some improvement in public health.

Interestingly, most interventions recruited young children, under the age of 13 years; perhaps as an effort to prevent excessive screen time and social media use in their later years, and to instill positive habits and long-term behavior change. Furthermore, a common observation of this review and previous systematic reviews is that a majority of the nondigital interventions targeting sedentary behavior and screen time are multicomponent and are often delivered through schools. Although this makes it difficult to evaluate the true effect of the screen time or sedentary behavior components, this observation suggests that addressing behavioral change in school-aged children and adolescents are most effective when

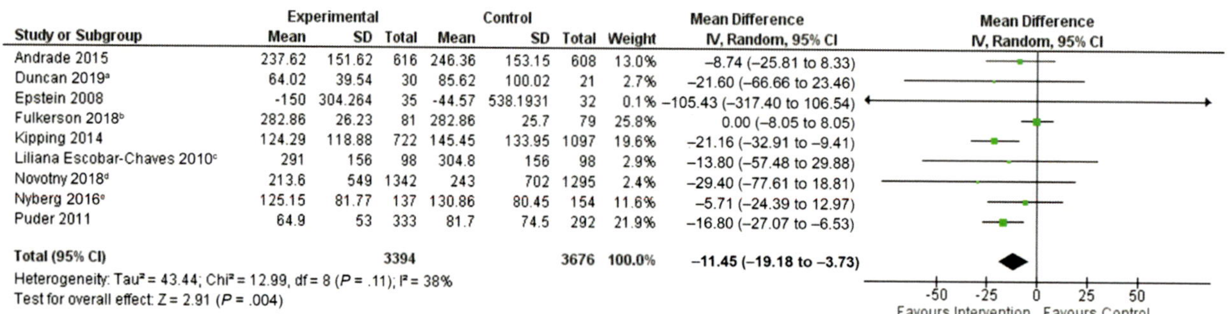

FIGURE 4

Forest plot of screen time all media (author defined; minutes per day). [a]Reported as hours per day, converted to minutes per day. [b]Reported as hours per week, converted to minutes per day. [c]Reported as hours per day, converted to minutes per day. [d]Reported as hours per day, converted to minutes per day. [e]Unpublished data, requested from author.

Study or Subgroup	Experimental Mean	Experimental SD	Experimental Total	Control Mean	Control SD	Control Total	Weight	Mean Difference IV, Random, 95% CI
Andrade 2015	18.46	46.41	616	20.08	47.82	608	29.0%	−1.62 (−6.90 to 3.66)
Jones 2008	38.04	53.2232	291	44.36	58.3917	315	19.5%	−6.32 (−15.21 to 2.57)
Liliana Escobar-Chaves 2010[a]	65.4	36	98	66.6	48	98	13.9%	−1.20 (−13.08 to 10.68)
Robinson 1999[b]	11.31	23.314	92	36.34	85.714	100	8.0%	−25.03 (−42.49 to −7.57)
Van Lippevelde 2014[c]	45	72.702	1569	43.8	72.906	1578	29.6%	1.20 (−3.89 to 6.29)
Total (95% CI)			**2666**			**2699**	**100.0%**	**−3.51 (−9.02 to 2.01)**

Heterogeneity: Tau² = 20.04; Chi² = 9.14, df = 4 (*P* = .06); I² = 56%
Test for overall effect: Z = 1.25 (*P* = .21)

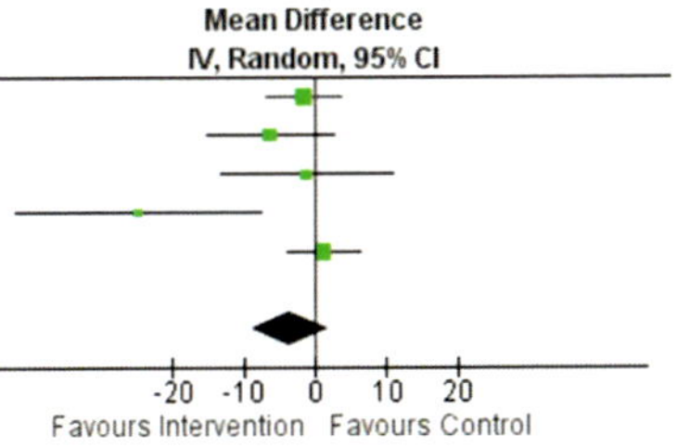

Mean Difference IV, Random, 95% CI: -20 -10 0 10 20; Favours Intervention Favours Control

FIGURE 5

Forest plot of screen time (author defined computer gaming or video games; minutes per day). [a]Reported as hours per day, converted to minutes per day. [b]Reported as hours per week, converted to minutes per day. [c]Reported as hours per day, converted to minutes per day.

used as a comprehensive and multifaceted strategy rather than a singular-component intervention. Similarly, school-based interventions alone may not be enough to counteract the trend of increasing screen time and sedentary behavior.

Although we included the largest number of studies to-date in a systematic review on screen time and sedentary behavior in SACA, most studies were conducted in HIC. It is possible that this finding is attributed to the stark inequality in digital connectivity in SACA living in LMIC. In the recent COVID-19 report, The International Telecommunication Union and United Nations Children's Fund (UNICEF) highlight that 1.2 billion children and adolescents (aged 3-17 years) do not have internet access at home, and primarily reside in South Asia, West, East, Central, or Southern Africa.[83] Likewise, disparities exist between HIC and LMIC in mobile phone ownership, although this gap is closing among youth. Physical inactivity, however, remains consistent across world regions.[11] Thus, as the world becomes more connected, we expect preventive interventions, policies, and programs to become more prevalent.

Unfortunately, this review and meta-analysis present similar gaps in the evidence and methodology as a previous scoping exercise of existing systematic reviews conducted by the authors. An overwhelming majority of interventions were implemented in high-income settings and the heterogeneity of available data because of diverse interventions, a lack of standardization of screen time metrics, vague and diverse methodologies, and use of subjective tools such as self-reported screen use limit the findings of this review. Thus, generalizability of these findings proves difficult. Furthermore, some of the findings of this review should be interpreted with caution, considering the quality of the evidence. Despite a robust number of studies included, very few were rated as high-quality. Moreover, although many studies reported a randomized-controlled design, the majority of included RCTs lacked description and/or implementation of more robust methods. Consistent with existing literature, the risk of bias in some areas was notable across the majority of studies; the most common risks of bias among included studies were failure to blind participants and personnel, attrition bias, and selective reporting. This limits and introduces a level of

Study or Subgroup	Experimental Mean	Experimental SD	Experimental Total	Control Mean	Control SD	Control Total	Weight	Mean Difference IV, Random, 95% CI
Foster 2008[a]	104.42	17.3647	269	108.93	17.3647	210	60.7%	−4.51 (−7.64 to −1.38)
Jones 2008	134.92	96.8935	291	151.91	105.602	315	2.3%	−16.99 (−33.11 to −0.87)
Kipping 2014	466.17	70.58	356	461.78	66.33	522	6.9%	4.39 (−4.89 to 13.67)
Lloyd 2018	764.5	43.29	359	766.36	39.98	386	16.6%	−1.86 (−7.86 to 4.14)
Novotny 2018	1,347.05	207.2808	1342	1,351.36	146.7474	1295	3.2%	−4.31 (−17.98 to 9.36)
Nyberg 2016[b]	316.06	46.33	122	320.46	40.8	114	4.8%	−4.40 (−15.52 to 6.72)
Robinson 1999[c]	228.6	159.6	92	243	271.8	100	0.2%	−14.40 (−76.86 to 48.06)
Van Lippevelde 2014[d]	506.4	133.08	1569	513	167.44	1578	5.3%	−6.60 (−17.16 to 3.96)
Total (95% CI)			**4400**			**4520**	**100.0%**	**−3.86 (−6.30 to −1.41)**

Heterogeneity: Tau² = 0.00; Chi² = 6.56, df = 7 (*P* = .48) ; I² = 0%
Test for overall effect: Z = 3.10 (*P* = .002)

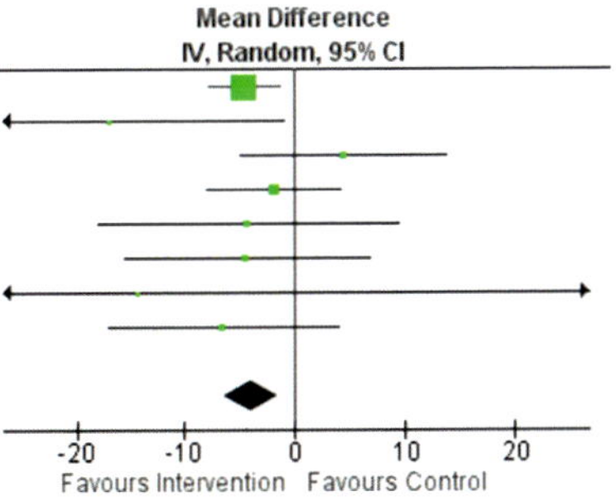

Mean Difference IV, Random, 95% CI: -20 -10 0 10 20; Favours Intervention Favours Control

FIGURE 6

Forest plot of sedentary behavior (author-defined; minutes per day). [a]Reported as hours per week, converted to minutes per day. [b]Unpublished data, requested from author. [c]Reported as hours per day, converted to minutes per day. [d]Reported as hours per day, converted to minutes per day.

Study or Subgroup	Experimental Mean	SD	Total	Control Mean	SD	Total	Weight	Mean Difference IV, Random, 95% CI
Jones 2008	70.68	60.2173	291	63.63	64.4261	315	3.0%	7.05 (−2.87 to 16.97)
Kipping 2014	54.39	21.55	424	56.65	23.42	649	24.2%	−2.26 (−4.99 to 0.47)
Lloyd 2018	57.99	22.34	359	56.98	19.39	386	21.4%	−1.01 (−2.00 to 4.02)
Novotny 2018	19.94	55.8351	1342	17.23	51.7285	1295	13.9%	2.71 (−1.40 to 6.82)
Nyberg 2016[a]	94.4	24.18	122	95.14	27.12	114	6.4%	−0.74 (−7.31 to 5.83)
Robinson 2010	-5.78	9.3	126	-4.88	7.71	117	31.1%	−0.90 (−3.04 to 1.24)
Total (95% CI)			**2664**			**2876**	**100.0%**	**−0.07 (−1.83 to 1.69)**

Heterogeneity: Tau² = 1.40; Chi² = 7.20, df = 5 (P = .21); I² = 31%
Test for overall effect: Z = 0.08 (P = .94)

FIGURE 7
Forest plot of moderate-to-vigorous physical activity (minutes per day). [a]Unpublished data, requested from author.

uncertainty regarding the efficacy of these types of interventions.

Implications for Policy, Recommendations and Research

With the rise of digital technologies, the proliferation of technology and connectivity have led to increased sedentary behaviors and poorer lifestyle behaviors in this age group. We know that increasingly poor lifestyle behaviors among youth and adolescents are no longer population health issues relegated to high-income settings. Thus, utilizing nondigital interventions to promote universal health, including physical activity and minimizing screen time are critical for long-term gains in human health and development. Future research should examine screen time as a proportion of sedentary time, as well as use standardized and objective measures of screen use and sedentary time. Policies and programs which reduce sedentary time and excessive screen use will be critical, especially in the post-COVID 19 reality.

ABBREVIATIONS

BMI: body mass index
CI: confidence interval
COVID-19: coronavirus disease 2019
HIC: high-income countries
LMIC: low- and middle-income countries
MD: mean difference
MVPA: moderate-to-vigorous physical activity
SACA: school-aged children and adolescents

FUNDING: This work was supported by a grant from the International Development Research Centre (#109010-001). The funder did not participate in the work. Core funding support was also provided by the SickKids Centre for Global Child Health in Toronto.

CONFLICT OF INTEREST DISCLOSURES: The authors have indicated they have no conflicts of interest to disclose.

REFERENCES

1. Felez-Nobrega M, Raine LB, Haro JM, Wijndaele K, Koyanagi A. Temporal trends in leisure-time sedentary behavior among adolescents aged 12-15 years from 26 countries in Asia, Africa, and the Americas. *Int J Behav Nutr Phys Act.* 2020;17(1):102
2. Reilly JJ, Kelly J. Long-term impact of overweight and obesity in childhood and adolescence on morbidity and premature mortality in adulthood: systematic review. *Int J Obes.* 2011; 35(7):891–898
3. Atkin AJ, Gorely T, Clemes SA, et al. Methods of measurement in epidemiology: sedentary behaviour. *Int J Epidemiol.* 2012;41(5):1460–1471
4. Stiglic N, Viner RM. Effects of screen-time on the health and well-being of children and adolescents: a systematic review of reviews. *BMJ Open.* 2019;9(1): e023191
5. Lapierre MA, Fleming-Milici F, Rozendaal E, McAlister AR, Castonguay J. The effect of advertising on children and adolescents. *Pediatrics.* 2017;140 (Suppl 2):S152–S156
6. Sadeghirad B, Duhaney T, Motaghipisheh S, Campbell NR, Johnston BC. Influence of unhealthy food and beverage marketing on children's dietary intake and preference: a systematic review and meta-analysis of randomized trials. *Obes Rev.* 2016;17(10): 945–959
7. Suchert V, Hanewinkel R, Isensee B. Sedentary behavior and indicators of mental health in school-aged children and adolescents: a systematic review. *Prev Med.* 2015;76:48–57
8. UNICEF. *The state of the world's children report. Children in a digital world.* Available at: https://www.unicef.org/reports/state-worlds-children-2017. Accessed March 29, 2021
9. Canadian Paediatric Society, Digital Health Task Force, Ottawa, Ontario.

Screen time and young children: promoting health and development in a digital world. *Paediatr Child Health.* 2017;22(8):461–468

10. Council on Communications and Media. Media use in school-aged children and adolescents. *Pediatrics.* 2016;138(5):e20162592
11. Guthold R, Stevens GA, Riley LM, Bull FC. Global trends in insufficient physical activity among adolescents: a pooled analysis of 298 population-based surveys with 1·6 million participants. *Lancet Child Adolesc Health.* 2020;4(1):23–35
12. Bates LC, Zieff G, Stanford K, et al. COVID-19 impact on behaviors across the 24-hour day in children and adolescents: physical activity, sedentary behavior, and sleep. *Children (Basel).* 2020;7(9):E138
13. Chaput JP, Willumsen J, Bull F, et al. 2020 WHO guidelines on physical activity and sedentary behaviour for children and adolescents aged 5-17 years: summary of the evidence. *Int J Behav Nutr Phys Act.* 2020;17(1):141
14. Alcântara CM, Silva ANS, Pinheiro PNDC, Queiroz MVO. Digital technologies for promotion of healthy eating habits in teenagers. *Rev Bras Enferm.* 2019; 72(2):513–520
15. Orben A, Przybylski AK. The association between adolescent well-being and digital technology use. *Nat Hum Behav.* 2019;3(2):173–182
16. Maniccia DM, Davison KK, Marshall SJ, Manganello JA, Dennison BA. A meta-analysis of interventions that target children's screen time for reduction. *Pediatrics.* 2011;128(1):e193–e210
17. Nguyen P, Le LK, Nguyen D, Gao L, Dunstan DW, Moodie M. The effectiveness of sedentary behaviour interventions on sitting time and screen time in children and adults: an umbrella review of systematic reviews. *Int J Behav Nutr Phys Act.* 2020;17(1):117
18. Wu L, Sun S, He Y, Jiang B. The effect of interventions targeting screen time reduction: a systematic review and meta-analysis. *Medicine (Baltimore).* 2016;95(27):e4029
19. van Grieken A, Ezendam NP, Paulis WD, van der Wouden JC, Raat H. Primary prevention of overweight in children and adolescents: a meta-analysis of the effectiveness of interventions aiming to decrease sedentary behaviour. *Int J Behav Nutr Phys Act.* 2012;9:61
20. Wahi G, Parkin PC, Beyene J, Uleryk EM, Birken CS. Effectiveness of interventions aimed at reducing screen time in children: a systematic review and meta-analysis of randomized controlled trials. *Arch Pediatr Adolesc Med.* 2011; 165(11):979–986
21. Biddle SJ, O'Connell S, Braithwaite RE. Sedentary behaviour interventions in young people: a meta-analysis. *Br J Sports Med.* 2011;45(11):937–942
22. Friedrich RR, Polet JP, Schuch I, Wagner MB. Effect of intervention programs in schools to reduce screen time: a meta-analysis. *J Pediatr (Rio J).* 2014; 90(3):232–241
23. Tremblay MS, LeBlanc AG, Kho ME, et al. Systematic review of sedentary behaviour and health indicators in school-aged children and youth. *Int J Behav Nutr Phys Act.* 2011;8(1):98
24. Oh C, Carducci B, Vaivada T, Bhutta ZA. Digital-based interventions for universal health promotion and health outcomes in school-aged children and adolescents: a systematic review and meta-analysis. *Pediatrics.* 2022;149(suppl 6): e2021053852H
25. Vaivada T, Oh C, Carducci B, Bhutta ZA. Rationale and approach to evaluating interventions to promote child health in LMICs. *Pediatrics.* 2022;149(suppl 6): e2021053852B
26. Higgins JPT, Thomas J, Chandler J, Cumpston M, Li T, Page MJ, Welch VA, eds. *Cochrane Handbook for Systematic Reviews of Interventions.* version 6.3 (updated February 2022). Available at: www.training.cochrane.org/handbook. Accessed March 29, 2021
27. Cochrane: Effective Practice and Organisation of Care. Summary assessments of the risk of bias. Available at: https://epoc.cochrane.org/sites/epoc.cochrane.org/files/public/uploads/Resources-for-authors2017/summary_assessments_of_the_risk_of_bias.pdf. Accessed March 29, 2021
28. Sterne JAC, Savović J, Page MJ, et al. RoB 2: a revised tool for assessing risk of bias in randomised trials. *BMJ.* 2019;366:l4898
29. Sterne JA, Hernán MA, Reeves BC, et al. ROBINS-I: a tool for assessing risk of bias in non-randomised studies of interventions. *BMJ.* 2016;355:i4919
30. Guyatt GH, Oxman AD, Vist GE, et al; GRADE Working Group. GRADE: an emerging consensus on rating quality of evidence and strength of recommendations. *BMJ.* 2008;336(7650):924–926
31. Kipping RR, Howe LD, Jago R, Campbell R, Wells S, Chittleboro CR, et al. Effect of intervention aimed at increasing physical activity, reducing sedentary behaviour, and increasing fruit and vegetable consumption in children: Active for Life Year 5 (AFLY5) school based cluster randomised controlled trial. *BMJ.* 2016; 348–g3256
32. Andrade S, Verloigne M, Cardon G, et al. School-based intervention on healthy behaviour among Ecuadorian adolescents: effect of a cluster-randomized controlled trial on screen-time. *BMC Public Health.* 2015;15(1):942
33. Aragon Neely J, Hudnut-Beumler J, White Webb M, et al. The effect of primary care interventions on children's media viewing habits and exposure to violence. *Acad Pediatr.* 2013;13(6):531–539
34. Colín-Ramírez E, Castillo-Martínez L, Orea-Tejeda A, Vergara-Castañeda A, Keirns-Davis C, Villa-Romero A. Outcomes of a school-based intervention (RESCATE) to improve physical activity patterns in Mexican children aged 8-10 years. *Health Educ Res.* 2010;25(6):1042–1049
35. Contento IR, Koch PA, Lee H, Calabrese-Barton A. Adolescents demonstrate improvement in obesity risk behaviors after completion of choice, control & change, a curriculum addressing personal agency and autonomous motivation. *J Am Diet Assoc.* 2010;110(12):1830–1839
36. Duncan S, Stewart T, McPhee J, et al. Efficacy of a compulsory homework programme for increasing physical activity and improving nutrition in children: a cluster randomised controlled trial. *Int J Behav Nutr Phys Act.* 2019;16(1):80
37. Epstein LH, Roemmich JN, Robinson JL, et al. A randomized trial of the effects of reducing television viewing and computer use on body mass index in young children. *Arch Pediatr Adolesc Med.* 2008;162(3):239–245
38. Escobar-Chaves SL, Markham CM, Addy RC, Greisinger A, Murray NG, Brehm B.

The fun families study: intervention to reduce children's TV viewing. *Obesity (Silver Spring)*. 2010;18(Suppl 1): S99–S101

39. Filho VCB, Bandeira ADS, Minatto G, et al. Effect of a multicomponent intervention on lifestyle factors among brazilian adolescents from low human development index areas: A cluster-randomized controlled trial. *Int J Environ Res Public Health*. 2019;16(2):267

40. Fulkerson JA, Friend S, Horning M, et al. Family home food environment and nutrition-related parent and child personal and behavioral outcomes of the healthy home offerings via the mealtime environment (HOME) plus program: a randomized controlled trial. *J Acad Nutr Diet*. 2018;118(2):240–251

41. Gentile DA, Welk G, Eisenmann JC, et al. Evaluation of a multiple ecological level child obesity prevention program: switch what you do, view, and chew. *BMC Med*. 2009;7:49

42. Habib-Mourad C, Ghandour LA, Maliha C, Awada N, Dagher M, Hwalla N. Impact of a one-year school-based teacher-implemented nutrition and physical activity intervention: main findings and future recommendations. *BMC Public Health*. 2020;20(1):256

43. Jones D, Hoelscher DM, Kelder SH, Hergenroeder A, Sharma SV. Increasing physical activity and decreasing sedentary activity in adolescent girls–the incorporating more physical activity and calcium in teens (IMPACT) study. *Int J Behav Nutr Phys Act*. 2008;5:42

44. Knebel MTG, Borgatto AF, Lopes MVV, et al. Mediating role of screen media use on adolescents' total sleep time: a cluster-randomized controlled trial for physical activity and sedentary behaviour. *Child Care Health Dev*. 2020;46(3):381–389

45. Kobel S, Lämmle C, Wartha O, Kesztyüs D, Wirt T, Steinacker JM. Effects of a randomised controlled school-based health promotion intervention on obesity related behavioural outcomes of children with migration background. *J Immigr Minor Health*. 2017;19(2):254–262

46. Lindenberg K, Halasy K, Schoenmaekers S. A randomized efficacy trial of a cognitive-behavioral group intervention to prevent internet use disorder onset in adolescents: the PROTECT study protocol. *Contemp Clin Trials Commun*. 2017;6: 64–71

47. Llargués E, Recasens A, Franco R, et al. Medium-term evaluation of an educational intervention on dietary and physical exercise habits in schoolchildren: the Avall 2 study. *Endocrinol Nutr*. 2012;59(5):288–295

48. Lloyd J, Creanor S, Logan S, et al. Effectiveness of the Healthy Lifestyles Programme (HeLP) to prevent obesity in UK primary-school children: a cluster randomised controlled trial. *Lancet Child Adolesc Health*. 2018;2(1):35–45

49. Novotny R, DAvis J, Butel J. Effect of the Children's Healthy Living Program on young child overweight, obesity, and acanthosis nigricans in the US-affiliated Pacific region: A randomized clinical trial.JAMA Netw Open. 2018;1(6):e183896

50. Nyberg G, Norman Å, Sundblom E, Zeebari Z, Elinder LS. Effectiveness of a universal parental support programme to promote health behaviours and prevent overweight and obesity in 6-year-old children in disadvantaged areas, the healthy school start study II, a cluster-randomised controlled trial. *Int J Behav Nutr Phys Act*. 2016;13:4

51. Puder JJ, Marques-Vidal P, Schindler C, et al. Effect of multidimensional lifestyle intervention on fitness and adiposity in predominantly migrant preschool children (Ballabeina): cluster randomised controlled trial. *BMJ*. 2011;343:d6195

52. Robinson TN, Matheson DM, Kraemer HC, et al. A randomized controlled trial of culturally tailored dance and reducing screen time to prevent weight gain in low-income African American girls: Stanford GEMS. *Arch Pediatr Adolesc Med*. 2010;164(11):995–1004

53. Robinson TN. Reducing children's television viewing to prevent obesity: a randomized controlled trial. *JAMA*. 1999;282(16):1561–1567

54. Sahota P, Rudolf MC, Dixey R, Hill AJ, Barth JH, Cade J. Randomised controlled trial of primary school based intervention to reduce risk factors for obesity. *BMJ*. 2001;323(7320):1029–1032

55. Salmon J, Ball K, Hume C, Booth M, Crawford D. Outcomes of a group-randomized trial to prevent excess weight gain, reduce screen behaviours and promote physical activity in 10-year-old children: switch-play. *Int J Obes*. 2008;32(4):601–612

56. Tarro L, Llauradó E, Aceves-Martins M, et al. Impact of a youth-led social marketing intervention run by adolescents to encourage healthy lifestyles among younger school peers (EYTO-Kids project): a parallel-cluster randomised controlled pilot study. *J Epidemiol Community Health*. 2019;73(4):324–333

57. Van Lippevelde W, Bere E, Verloigne M, et al. The role of family-related factors in the effects of the UP4FUN school-based family-focused intervention targeting screen time in 10- to 12-year-old children: the ENERGY project. *BMC Public Health*. 2014;14:857

58. Wang Y, Tussing L, Odoms-Young A, et al. Obesity prevention in low socioeconomic status urban African-American adolescents: study design and preliminary findings of the HEALTH-KIDS Study. *Eur J Clin Nutr*. 2006;60(1):92–103

59. Xu F, Wang X, Ware RS, et al. A school-based comprehensive lifestyle intervention among Chinese kids against obesity (CLICK-Obesity) in Nanjing City, China: the baseline data. *Asia Pac J Clin Nutr*. 2014;23(1):48–54

60. Foster GD, Sherman S, Borradaile KE, et al. A policy-based school intervention to prevent overweight and obesity. *Pediatrics*. 2008;121(4):e794–e802

61. Neumark-Sztainer DR, Friend SE, Flattum CF, et al. New moves-preventing weight-related problems in adolescent girls a group-randomized study. *Am J Prev Med*. 2010;39(5):421–432

62. Simon C, Wagner A, Platat C, et al. ICAPS: a multilevel program to improve physical activity in adolescents. Diabetes Metab. 2006;32(1):41

63. Spruijt-Metz D, Nguyen-Michel ST, Goran MI, Chou CP, Huang TT. Reducing sedentary behavior in minority girls via a theory-based, tailored classroom media intervention. *Int J Pediatr Obes*. 2008; 3(4):240–248

64. Salmon J, Arundell L, Hume C, et al. A cluster-randomized controlled trial to reduce sedentary behavior and promote physical activity and health of 8-9 year olds: the transform-us! study. *BMC Public Health*. 2011;11:759

65. Salway R, Sebire SJ, Tibbitts B, et al. Physical activity and psychosocial

characteristics of the peer supporters in the PLAN-A study-a latent class analysis. *Int J Environ Res Public Health.* 2020;17(21): 7980

66. Morgan PJ, Young MD, Barnes AT, Eather N, Pollock ER, Lubans DR. Engaging fathers to increase physical activity in girls: the "Dads And Daughters Exercising and Empowered" (DADEE) randomized controlled trial. *Ann Behav Med.* 2019;53(1):39–52
67. Veldman SLC, Jones RA, Stanley RM, et al. Promoting physical activity and executive functions among children: a cluster randomized controlled trial of an after-school program in Australia. *J Phys Act Health.* 2020;17(10):940–946
68. van Nassau F, Singh AS, Cerin E, et al. The Dutch obesity intervention in teenagers (DOiT) cluster controlled implementation trial: intervention effects and mediators and moderators of adiposity and energy balance-related behaviours. *Int J Behav Nutr Phys Act.* 2014;11:158
69. Verbestel V, De Henauw S, Barba G, et al; IDEFICS consortium. Effectiveness of the IDEFICS intervention on objectively measured physical activity and sedentary time in European children. *Obes Rev.* 2015;16(suppl 2):57–67
70. Cronholm F, Rosengren BE, Karlsson C, Karlsson MK. A comparative study found that a seven-year school-based exercise programme increased physical activity levels in both sexes. *Acta Paediatr.* 2018;107(4):701–707
71. Schmidt SK, Reinboth MS, Resaland GK, Bratland-Sanda S. Changes in physical activity, physical fitness and well-being following a school-based health promotion program in a Norwegian region with a poor public health profile: a non-randomized controlled study in early adolescents. *Int J Environ Res Public Health.* 2020;17(3):E896
72. Bickham DS, Hswen Y, Slaby RG, Rich M. A preliminary evaluation of a school-based media education and reduction intervention. *J Prim Prev.* 2018;39(3): 229–245
73. Breslin G, Brennan D, Rafferty R, Gallagher AM, Hanna D. The effect of a healthy lifestyle programme on 8-9 year olds from social disadvantage. *Arch Dis Child.* 2012;97(7):618–624
74. Cong Z, Feng D, Liu Y, Esperat MC. Sedentary behaviors among Hispanic children: influences of parental support in a school intervention program. *Am J Health Promot.* 2012;26(5):270–280
75. Gholamian B, Shahnazi H, Hassanzadeh A. The effect of educational intervention based on BASNEF model for reducing internet addiction among female students: a quasi-experimental study. *Ital J Pediatr.* 2019;45(1):164
76. Harrison M, Burns CF, McGuinness M, Heslin J, Murphy NM. Influence of a health education intervention on physical activity and screen time in primary school children: 'Switch Off–Get Active'. *J Sci Med Sport.* 2006;9(5):388–394
77. Murillo Pardo B, García Bengoechea E, Generelo Lanaspa E, Zaragoza Casterad J, Julián Clemente JA. Effects of the 3-year Sigue la Huella intervention on sedentary time in secondary school students. *Eur J Public Health.* 2015;25(3):438–443
78. Racine EF, DeBate RD, Gabriel KP, High RR. The relationship between media use and psychological and physical assets among third- to fifth-grade girls. *J Sch Health.* 2011;81(12):749–755
79. Van Kann DH, de Vries SI, Schipperijn J, de Vries NK, Jansen MW, Kremers SP. A multicomponent schoolyard intervention targeting children's recess physical activity and sedentary behavior: effects after one year [published online ahead of print October 24, 2016] [retraction appears in *J Phys Act Health.* 2017;14(5):416]. *J Phys Act Health.* doi: 10.1123/jpah.2015-0702.
80. van Stralen MM, de Meij J, Te Velde SJ, et al. Mediators of the effect of the JUMP-in intervention on physical activity and sedentary behavior in Dutch primary schoolchildren from disadvantaged neighborhoods. *Int J Behav Nutr Phys Act.* 2012;9:131–142
81. Sevil J, García-González L, Abós Á, Generelo E, Aibar A. Can high schools be an effective setting to promote healthy lifestyles? Effects of a multiple behavior change intervention in adolescents. *J Adolesc Health.* 2019;64(4):478–486
82. Shukri M, Zin Z, Zainol K, Said S, Rajali A. The effectiveness of a computer-based method to support eating intervention among economically disadvantaged children in Malaysia. *Health Educ J.* 2019;78(5):497–509
83. United Nations Children's Fund and International Telecommunication Union. *How many children and young people have internet access at home? Estimating digital connectivity during the COVID-19 pandemic.* Available at: https://data.unicef.org/resources/children-and-young-people-internet-access-at-home-during-covid19/#:~:text=Globally%2C%20only%2033%20per%20cent,have%20internet%20access%20at%20home. Accessed March 29, 2021

Trends in Adolescent Online and Offline Victimization and Suicide Risk Factors

Noah T. Kreski, MPH,[a] Qixuan Chen, PhD,[b] Mark Olfson, MD, MPH,[a,c] Magdalena Cerdá, DrPH,[d] Deborah Hasin, PhD,[a,c] Silvia S. Martins, MD, PhD,[a] Pia M. Mauro, PhD,[a] Katherine M. Keyes, PhD[a]

abstract

OBJECTIVE: Suicidal ideation and plans are increasing among US adolescents. Changing prevalence of online victimization is frequently hypothesized as an explanation for this increase. We tested trends in online and offline victimization and whether they contribute to recent trends in adolescent suicidal outcomes.

METHODS: Youth Risk Behavior Survey data (2011–2019, $N = 73\,074$) were collected biennially through national cross-sectional surveys of US school-attending adolescents. We examined trends in past-year victimization. We also examined whether the relationship between victimization and past-year suicidal ideation, plans, attempts, and injury changed over time using survey-weighted logistic regressions that adjusted for sex and race and ethnicity. We also sex-stratified results to examine sex differences.

RESULTS: Although suicidal ideation and plans increased among US adolescents (mainly girls), online and offline victimization prevalence did not increase over time (offline: 20.0% in 2011, 19.5% in 2019; online: 16.2% in 2011, 15.7% in 2019). Online and offline victimization were associated with suicidal outcomes, especially co-occurring online and offline victimization (eg, adjusted odds ratio [co-occurring online and offline victimization versus none, outcome: suicidal injury] = 8.37; 95% confidence interval: 7.06–9.91). The magnitude of the associations between victimization and suicidal outcomes largely remained stable over time.

CONCLUSION: Peer victimization prevalence has not sufficiently changed over time in concert with suicidal outcomes to explain increased suicidal outcomes. The prevalence of victimization has remained relatively invariant across time despite growing awareness and programming, making online and offline victimization consistent, socially-patterned risk factors that warrant further monitoring and interventions. Research must examine risk factors beyond victimization to explain increasing suicidal outcomes.

Full article can be found online at www.pediatrics.org/cgi/doi/10.1542/peds.2020-049585

[a]Departments of Epidemiology and [b]Biostatistics, Mailman School of Public Health, Columbia University, New York, New York; [c]Department of Psychiatry, New York State Psychiatric Institute, Vagelos College of Physicians and Surgeons, Columbia University Irving Medical Center, New York, New York; and [d]Department of Population Health, School of Medicine, New York University, New York, New York

Mx. Kreski conducted the analyses, drafted the initial text of the manuscript, and contributed all tables and figures, as well as incorporated coauthor feedback; Dr Keyes conceptualized the study and analyses, as well as critically reviewed and revised the manuscript; Drs Chen, Olfson, Cerdá, Hasin, Martins, and Mauro critically reviewed the manuscript for important intellectual content, interpreted data, and provided direct edits and feedback to strengthen the text; and all authors approved the final manuscript as submitted and agree to be accountable for all aspects of the work.

DOI: https://doi.org/10.1542/peds.2020-049585

Accepted for publication May 14, 2021

WHAT'S KNOWN ON THE SUBJECT: Bullying victimization is linked to worse adolescent mental health, which is an urgent priority given increases in US adolescent suicidality.

WHAT THIS STUDY ADDS: Although the links between victimization and suicidal behavior are clear, victimization is not changing, either in prevalence or in the strength of the association with suicidality, over time to explain suicidal behavior trends.

To cite: Kreski NT, Chen Q, Olfson M, et al. Trends in Adolescent Online and Offline Victimization and Suicide Risk Factors. *Pediatrics.* 2021;148(3):e2020049585

ARTICLE

Suicidal behavior in children and adolescents is an increasingly serious problem, with 3000 suicide deaths among youth ages 10 to 19 in 2018.[1] The national number of emergency department visits by children and adolescents with suicide attempts and ideation nearly doubled between 2007 and 2015,[2] and suicide deaths among youth ages 10 to 19 increased from 4.37 to 7.10 per 100 000 between 2009 and 2018.[1] Data from the Youth Risk Behavior Survey (YRBS) indicate that suicidal ideation and plans have increased among US adolescents since 2009, with significant heterogeneity by sex, given that trends were primarily seen among female adolescents.[3–5] Understanding the factors behind these trends is an important public health issue.

One factor hypothesized to contribute to recent trends in adolescent suicide is peer victimization, partially in person (ie, perceived offline victimization) but especially through the rise of social media and other Internet sites (ie, perceived online victimization).[6] Offline[7,8] and online bullying and victimization[7,9] are well-documented as factors associated with adolescent mental health and suicidal outcomes.[10] They are also correlated with each other,[11,12] indicating that adolescents who are victimized online are more likely to be victimized offline as well.

Although researchers in previous studies have demonstrated a link between peer victimization and adverse psychiatric outcomes, much remains unknown. Specific questions include whether the prevalence of peer victimization has changed, whether such trends in peer victimization explain increases in suicidal outcomes, and whether these dynamics apply equally across sexes. Online and offline peer victimization could explain trends in suicidal ideation, plans, attempts, and injury among adolescents if their prevalence had increased in concert with the prevalence of these suicidal outcomes. Although opportunities for anonymous online interaction (and thus victimization) have increased with the proliferation of social media and other online engagement sources, it is not known whether these opportunities have translated to changes in peer victimization prevalence. Online and offline peer victimization may also explain trends in suicidal outcomes if the magnitude of the relationship between victimization and a given outcome has increased over time, yet no studies to date have assessed time trends in the magnitude of these risk factor relationships, overall or by sex.

In this study, we aimed to examine (1) whether online or offline peer victimization and suicidal ideation, plans, attempts, and injury have increased in prevalence over time, and (2) the extent to which victimization explains trends in suicidal outcomes within a US nationally representative sample of adolescents from 2011 to 2019, overall and by sex. Findings could be used to inform suicide prevention interventions, adding nuanced understanding of the specific risks posed by various forms of victimization and exploring

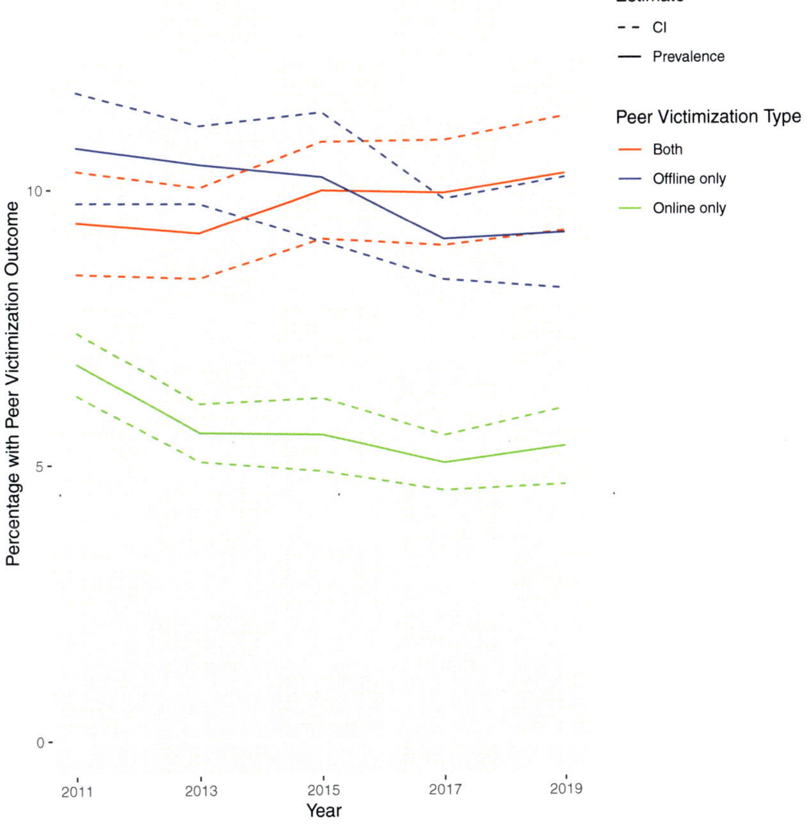

FIGURE 1

Trends in peer victimization among high school students, 2011–2019 YRBS. Offline victimization was assessed with the question: "During the past 12 months, have you ever been bullied on school property?"; Online victimization was assessed with the question: "During the past 12 months, have you ever been electronically bullied? (Count being bullied through texting, Instagram, Facebook, or other social media.)."

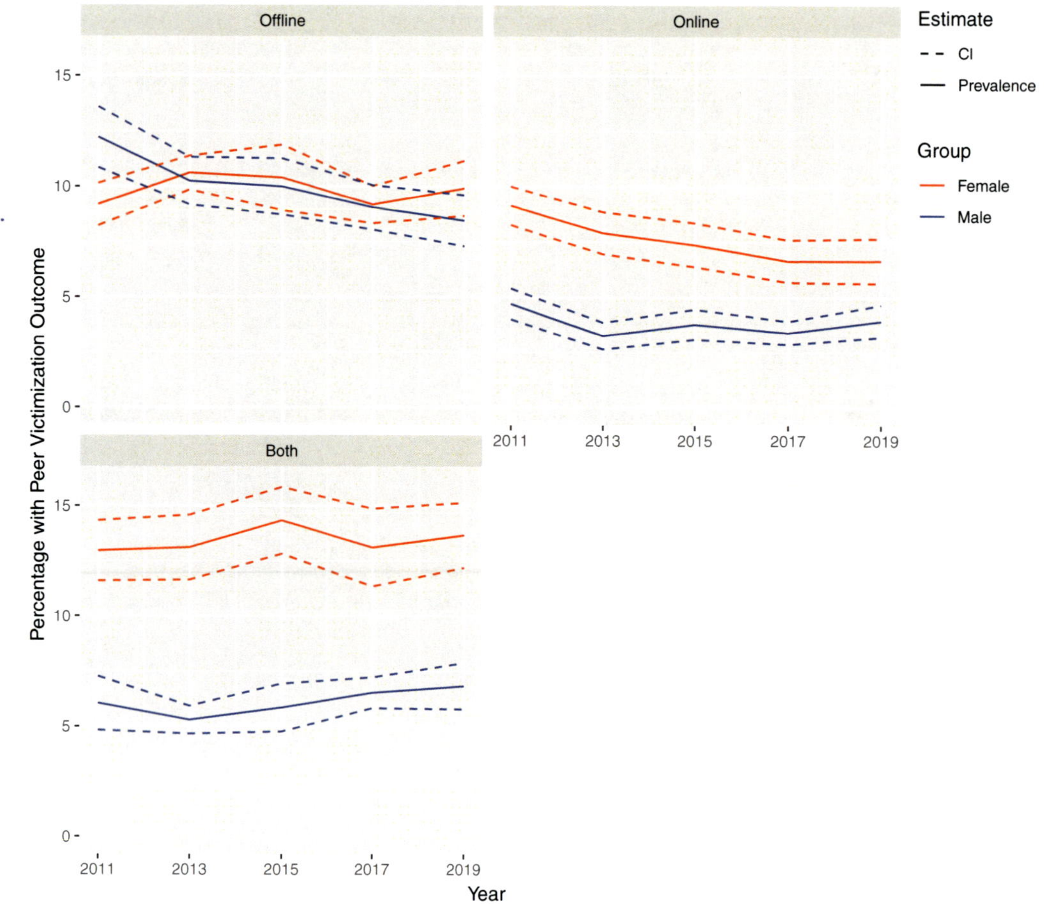

FIGURE 2
Trends in peer victimization among high school students, split by sex, 2011–2019 YRBS.

the extent to which trends in suicidal outcomes are accounted for by victimization.

METHODS

We used YRBS data collected biennially through national cross-sectional surveys, with ~15 000 US school-attending adolescents in each survey (grades 9 to 12). Participation is voluntary and anonymous. As of 2019, the school response rate was 75.1%, whereas the student response rate was 80.3%.[13] The Centers for Disease Control and Prevention Institutional Review Board approved the protocol. Full sample size was 73 074 from 2011 to 2019, starting with the year when online victimization was introduced to the survey.

Measures

The YRBS included 4 items related to suicide. Suicidal ideation was assessed with the question, "During the past 12 months, did you ever seriously consider attempting suicide?" Suicide plans were assessed with the question, "During the past 12 months, did you make a plan about how you would attempt suicide?" Suicide attempts were assessed with the question, "During the past 12 months, how many times did you actually attempt suicide?" Suicide injury was assessed with the question, "If you attempted suicide during the past 12 months, did any attempt result in an injury, poisoning, or overdose that had to be treated by a doctor or nurse?". Items that queried the number of times in which suicidal behavior occurred were dichotomized into any versus none. These items exhibit strong convergent and discriminant validity.[14]

Perceived peer victimization was assessed with 2 self-reported items with yes or no responses. Offline victimization was assessed with the question "During the past 12 months, have you ever been bullied on school property?" Online victimization was assessed with the

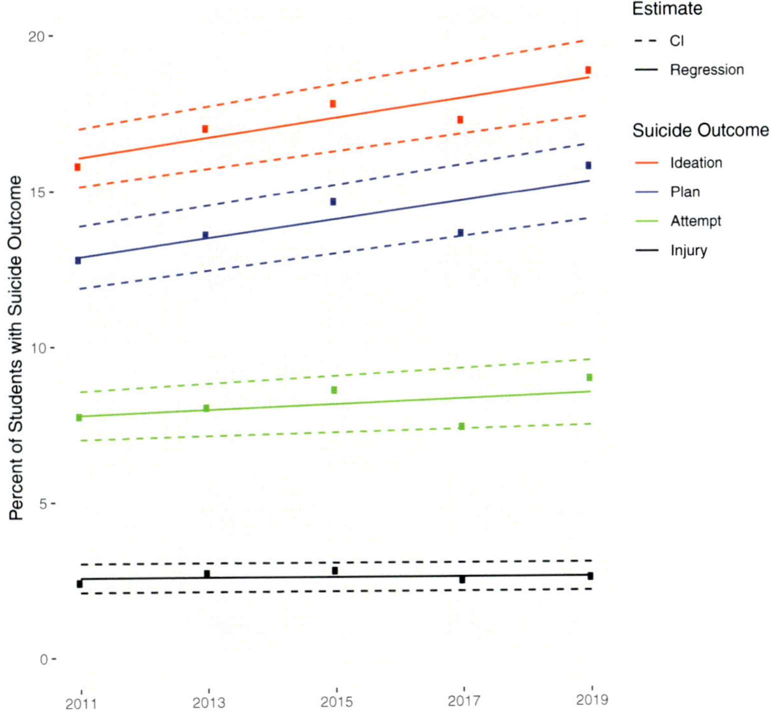

FIGURE 3
Trends in suicide outcomes, 2011–2019 YRBS. Plan: During the past 12 months, did you make a plan about how you would attempt suicide? Attempt: During the past 12 months, how many times did you actually attempt suicide? Injury: If you attempted suicide during the past 12 months, did any attempt result in an injury, poisoning, or overdose that had to be treated by a doctor or nurse?

question "During the past 12 months, have you ever been electronically bullied? (Count being bullied through texting, Instagram, Facebook, or other social media.)" These items were combined into a four-level exposure from 2011 onward: no victimization, online only, offline only, or both online and offline.

To account for potential demographic confounding, we examined sex and race and ethnicity as covariates. Sex was self-described as "male" or "female," and race and ethnicity were based on 5 self-reported categories, with options to select as many as applicable, and reconfigured into 6 categories: American Indian or Alaskan Native, Asian American and Pacific Islander, non-Hispanic Black or African American, Hispanic and/or Latino, non-Hispanic white, and non-Hispanic multiracial.

Race and ethnicity are examined here as a social construct and important personal identity which, along with sex, can shape both peer victimization experiences and suicidal outcomes. For instance, adolescents of color can face uniquely harmful effects of bias-based peer victimization, or disproportionate levels of contextual-level risk factors linked to peer victimization (eg, adverse school environments).[15] For suicidal outcomes, not only do the factors contributing to suicidal behavior vary across racial and ethnic categories,[16] but the prevalence of these outcomes varied across racial and ethnic groups in YRBS data.[17] These prevalence disparities also occurred by sex, with girls having higher levels of both suicidal outcomes and peer victimization.[17,18] Therefore, controlling for this racial, ethnic, and sexual heterogeneity is an important step needed to understand the extent to which peer victimization explains and predicts suicidal outcomes at the population level.

Statistical analysis

We estimated prevalence and 95% confidence intervals (CIs) of offline only, online only, and co-occurring forms of victimization in each biennial YRBS survey. We also estimated the biyearly time trends in victimization using survey-weighted logistic regression models with each form of victimization as the outcome and the continuous year (per 2 years) as a predictor.

We characterized trends in suicidal outcomes with the biennial prevalence estimates and 95% CIs of dichotomous self-reported outcomes (ideation, plans, attempts, injury).

To examine the extent to which victimization predicts each outcome, we fit separate survey-weighted logistic regression models to assess the association between each form of victimization and each of the 4 binary suicide outcomes, unadjusted and adjusted for sex and race and ethnicity.

To further understand whether victimization explains trends in suicidal outcomes, we compared estimates for year predicting each outcome with and without adjustment for victimization. Additionally, we examined temporal heterogeneity in the association between victimization and suicidal outcomes by fitting weighted logistic regression models linking victimization and each outcome for each survey year and testing whether associations vary over time by including the interaction between year (treated categorically) and victimization in models using data from all survey years.

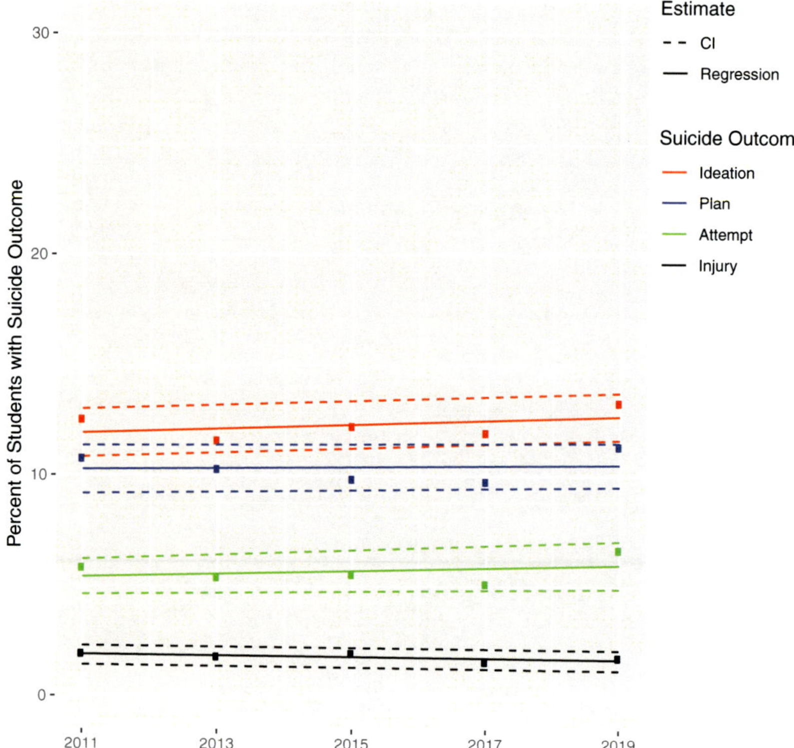

FIGURE 4

Trends in suicide outcomes, male, 2011–2019 YRBS. Plan: During the past 12 months, did you make a plan about how you would attempt suicide? Attempt: During the past 12 months, how many times did you actually attempt suicide? Injury: If you attempted suicide during the past 12 months, did any attempt result in an injury, poisoning, or overdose that had to be treated by a doctor or nurse?

Finally, to examine heterogeneity by sex in these associations and patterns, we stratified all of the above analyses by sex. Sample sizes for many racial and ethnic groups were too small to have sufficient power for stratification.

We used the SURVEYFREQ procedure (SAS 9.4; SAS Institute, Inc, Cary, NC) to estimate prevalence and the SURVEYLOGISTIC procedure (SAS 9.4) to fit logistic regression models. All statistical analyses accounted for the complex sampling design with YRBS.

RESULTS

Distributions of demographic variables, experiences of victimization, and suicidal outcomes by year can be seen in Supplemental Table 6.

Trends in Offline and Online Victimization

In 2019, 24.78% of participants reported any victimization, whereas the overall prevalence of experiencing victimization over the study period was consistently close to the overall mean of 25.35%. The prevalence of offline and online victimization stayed relatively flat over the study period (Fig 1), with slight decreases in the experience of offline only or online only victimization over time (odds ratio [OR] for each 2-year increase in time = 0.98 [95% CI: 0.96–0.99] and 0.97 [95% CI: 0.95–0.99], respectively). Co-occurring online and offline victimization increased from 9.4% in 2011% to 10.3% in 2019, but there was limited evidence for trends (OR for each 2-year increase in time = 1.01 [95% CI: 1.00–1.03; $P > .05$]). Victimization experiences were correlated; students who experienced offline victimization had 12.95 times the odds of experiencing online victimization compared with students who did not (95% CI: 12.03–13.95).

By sex, patterns were relatively consistent, although disparities existed (Fig 2). Offline only victimization decreased for male adolescents and was static for female adolescents (OR for each 2-year increase in time = 0.95 [95% CI–0.93, 0.97] and 1.00 [95% CI: 0.98–1.02], respectively). Conversely, online only victimization was static for male adolescents and decreased for female adolescents (OR for each 2-year increase in time = 0.98 [95% CI: 0.95–1.01] and 0.96 [95% CI: 0.94–0.98]). For male and female adolescents, co-occurring online and offline victimization prevalence has remained stable (OR for each 2-year increase in time = 1.02 [95% CI: 0.99–1.06] and 1.01 [95% CI: 0.99–1.03] respectively).

Trends in Suicidal Outcomes

Suicidal ideation prevalence gradually increased from 2011 (15.8%) to 2019 (18.8%). Similar trends emerged for making suicide plans, but trends for reported suicide attempts or injury by attempt were less marked (Fig 3). Suicidal ideation and plans were not increasing for male adolescents (Fig 4), but they were for female adolescents (Fig 5), and all outcomes were higher for female adolescents.

Associations Between Offline and Online Victimization and Suicidal Outcomes

The relationships between each form of victimization and suicidal outcomes are displayed in Table 1, which includes the unadjusted associations and the associations

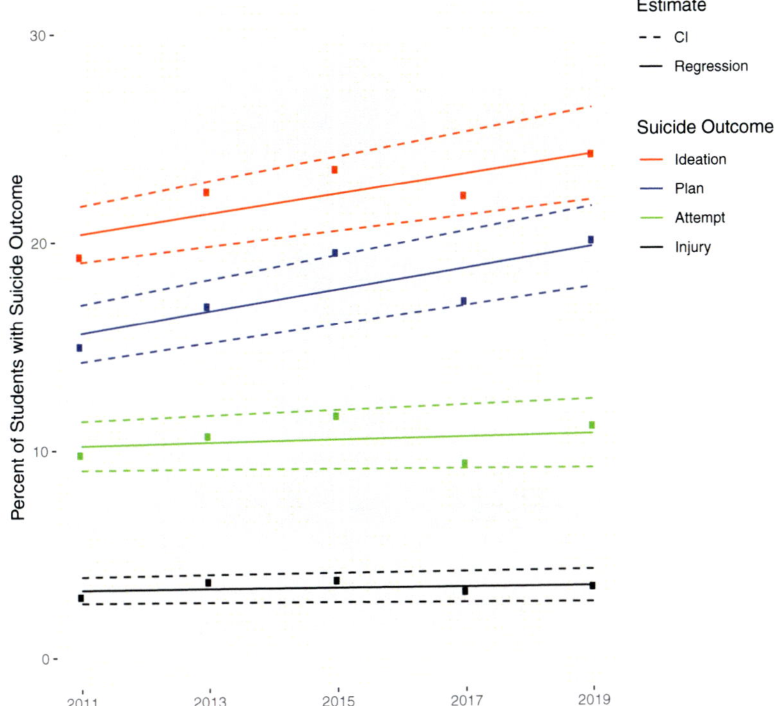

FIGURE 5

Trends in suicide outcomes, female, 2011–2019 YRBS. Plan: During the past 12 months, did you make a plan about how you would attempt suicide? Attempt: During the past 12 months, how many times did you actually attempt suicide? Injury: If you attempted suicide during the past 12 months, did any attempt result in an injury, poisoning, or overdose that had to be treated by a doctor or nurse?

adjusting for sex and race and ethnicity. Experiences of online only, offline only, and co-occurring victimization were all associated with each of the 4 suicidal outcomes. After adjustment, the associations between victimization and suicidal outcomes ranged in magnitude from the association between online victimization and having suicidal plans (adjusted odds ratio [aOR] = 2.69, 95% CI: 2.40–3.02) to the association between co-occurring online and offline victimization and suicidal injury (aOR = 8.37, 95% CI: 7.06–9.91).

There was some heterogeneity in the links between victimization and suicidal outcomes by sex, particularly for suicidal plans, attempts, and injury (Table 2). Whereas links between offline victimization and these outcomes were relatively consistent between sexes, links between online or co-occurring patterns of victimization and these outcomes were stronger for male adolescents.

Offline and Online Victimization Explaining Trends in Suicidal Outcomes

Adjusting for victimization increased, rather than decreased, the model estimate for year predicting the outcome of suicidal ideation (unadjusted β: 0.0199 versus adjusted β: 0.0236), suicide plans (unadjusted β: 0.0231 versus adjusted β: 0.0264), suicide attempts (unadjusted β: 0.0126 versus adjusted β: 0.0143), and suicidal injury (unadjusted β: 0.00466 versus adjusted β: 0.00567). The regression coefficients, β, can be interpreted as the increase in log odds of each suicide outcome given a 2-year increase. For both suicidal ideation and plans, the significantly increasing trends remained significant after adjustment for victimization (aOR for each 2-year increase in time [suicidal ideation] = 1.02, 95% CI: 1.01–1.04; [suicidal plans] = 1.03, 95% CI: 1.01–1.04). By sex, patterns were similar, as adjusting for victimization did not decrease the model estimate for year predicting each outcome for either male or female adolescents.

TABLE 1 Unadjusted ORs and aORs for Suicide Outcomes Based on Experiences of Victimization (Reference = No Victimization), 2011–2019 YRBS

	Experience of Victimization		
Suicidal Behavior Outcome	Offline Victimization Only	Online Victimization Only	Both
Suicidal ideation, OR (95% CI)	2.83 (2.61–3.07)	3.11 (2.81–3.45)	6.40 (5.92–6.92)
Suicidal ideation,[a] aOR (95% CI)	2.84 (2.62–3.07)	2.83 (2.55–3.14)	5.83 (5.37–6.32)
Suicidal plans, OR (95% CI)	2.71 (2.48–2.96)	2.88 (2.58–3.21)	5.78 (5.29–6.33)
Suicidal plans,[a] aOR (95% CI)	2.76 (2.53–3.01)	2.69 (2.40–3.02)	5.40 (4.92–5.92)
Suicide attempts, OR (95% CI)	2.74 (2.42–3.09)	3.58 (3.13–4.08)	6.84 (6.14–7.63)
Suicide attempts,[a] aOR (95% CI)	2.83 (2.51–3.21)	3.42 (2.98–3.92)	6.81 (6.08–7.62)
Suicide injury, OR (95% CI)	2.67 (2.19–3.25)	4.39 (3.53–5.46)	8.10 (6.89–9.53)
Suicide injury,[a] aOR (95% CI)	2.79 (2.28–3.41)	4.32 (3.40–5.48)	8.37 (7.06–9.91)

[a]Adjusted for race and ethnicity and sex.

TABLE 2 Unadjusted ORs and aORs for Suicide Outcomes Based on Experiences of Victimization (Reference = No Victimization), by Sex, 2011–2019 YRBS

Suicidal Behavior Outcome	Female			Male			Interaction *P*
	Offline Victimization Only	Online Victimization Only	Both	Offline Victimization Only	Online Victimization Only	Both	
Suicidal ideation, OR (95% CI)	2.81 (2.55–3.09)	2.68 (2.38–3.02)	5.44 (4.93–6.02)	2.84 (2.50–3.23)	3.12 (2.56–3.81)	6.50 (5.71–7.39)	.1378
Suicidal ideation,[a] aOR (95% CI)	2.85 (2.58–3.15)	2.73 (2.42–3.08)	5.68 (5.11–6.30)	2.80 (2.46–3.19)	3.08 (2.52–3.75)	6.30 (5.54–7.16)	
Suicidal plans, OR (95% CI)	2.72 (2.45–3.03)	2.40 (2.12–2.73)	4.86 (4.37–5.40)	2.65 (2.31–3.04)	3.21 (2.61–3.94)	6.23 (5.34–7.27)	.0070
Suicidal plans,[a] aOR (95% CI)	2.80 (2.52–3.12)	2.49 (2.18–2.83)	5.14 (4.60–5.74)	2.68 (2.33–3.08)	3.22 (2.62–3.95)	6.11 (5.23–7.14)	
Suicide attempts, OR (95% CI)	2.74 (2.38–3.17)	2.83 (2.40–3.33)	5.70 (5.02–6.46)	2.64 (2.15–3.23)	4.53 (3.50–5.84)	7.35 (6.13–8.81)	.0015
Suicide attempts,[a] aOR (95% CI)	2.86 (2.48–3.30)	2.98 (2.52–3.51)	6.43 (5.66–7.31)	2.78 (2.26–3.42)	4.64 (3.59–6.00)	7.70 (6.33–9.36)	
Suicide injury, OR (95% CI)	2.59 (1.99–3.38)	3.33 (2.57–4.32)	6.78 (5.60–8.22)	2.72 (1.96–3.80)	6.20 (4.13–9.29)	8.81 (6.67–11.64)	.0459
Suicide injury,[a] aOR (95% CI)	2.70 (2.08–3.51)	3.52 (2.69–4.62)	7.53 (6.21–9.13)	2.92 (2.09–4.07)	6.40 (4.21–9.71)	9.85 (7.36–13.19)	—

—, not applicable.

[a]Adjusted for race and ethnicity.

Offline and Online Victimization Predicting Suicidal Outcomes Over Time

In Table 3 we characterize the association between each form of victimization and each suicidal outcome in each time point adjusting for sex and race and ethnicity, as well as the *P* values testing the interactions between victimization and year predicting each outcome. The interactions between year and online only victimization indicated no substantial changes in the magnitude of associations across time. The same was found for offline only victimization. However, the association between co-occurring online and offline victimization and suicidal injury has generally changed over time (eg, 2011 aOR = 4.33 [95% CI: 2.77–6.76]; 2019 aOR = 7.66 [95% CI: 5.08–11.55]). Similar patterns were observed in the unadjusted models (Supplemental Table 7).

In Tables 4 and 5 we characterize these associations over time by sex. For female adolescents (Table 4), the interactions between year and each form of victimization indicated no substantial changes in the magnitude of associations across time (all *P* values > 0.05). For male adolescents (Table 5), although there were combinations of victimization pattern and suicidal outcome that exhibited heterogeneity in the strength of associations over time, these changes were not monotonic, and male suicidal outcomes exhibited no significant increases since 2011.

DISCUSSION

This study aimed to estimate the extent to which victimization explained trends in adolescent suicidal outcomes, overall and by sex. For victimization to explain increases in a given outcome, victimization would need to be increasing over time or the strength of the association between victimization and a given suicidal outcome would need to increase over time, but neither situation occurred for the general population, nor did either dynamic apply to male or female adolescents. Victimization has remained relatively stable in prevalence over time, whereas suicidal outcomes, particularly ideation and plans, have increased from 2011 onward (specifically among female adolescents). Although there is a strong relationship between peer victimization and suicidal outcomes, the only heterogeneity in the strength of the association between victimization and a specific outcome in the overall population was observed for co-occurring online and offline victimization and suicidal injury, which is not increasing over time (OR for suicidal injury per 2-year time point: 1.01, 95% CI: 0.98–1.03). Additionally, if peer victimization were contributing to increasing suicidal outcome trends, then the model estimate for year predicting a given outcome should reduce after adjustment for victimization. However, this was not the case for any of the suicidal outcomes.

TABLE 3 aORs for Suicide Outcomes Based on Experiences of Victimization by Year, 2011–2019 YRBS

Victimization Experience Predictor, Suicidal Behavior Outcome	2011, aOR (95% CI)	2013, aOR (95% CI)	2015, aOR (95% CI)	2017, aOR (95% CI)	2019, aOR (95% CI)	*P* For Interaction Between Year and Victimization
Offline Victimization (reference: none)						
Suicidal ideation	2.65 (2.24–3.13)	2.85 (2.36–3.45)	2.92 (2.57–3.32)	3.12 (2.62–3.72)	2.66 (2.15–3.29)	.7502
Suicidal plans	2.70 (2.26–3.23)	2.72 (2.35–3.17)	2.37 (1.96–2.86)	3.26 (2.68–3.97)	2.84 (2.26–3.57)	.2337
Suicide attempts	2.33 (1.82–2.99)	2.82 (2.29–3.47)	2.83 (2.09–3.84)	3.64 (2.84–4.66)	2.66 (1.98–3.58)	.2361
Suicide injury	1.67 (1.01–2.76)	2.88 (2.05–4.06)	3.19 (2.10–4.86)	4.15 (2.80–6.15)	2.31 (1.30–4.11)	.0868
Online victimization (reference: none)						
Suicidal ideation	3.26 (2.65–4.01)	2.86 (2.27–3.59)	2.58 (2.08–3.20)	3.40 (2.69–4.30)	2.21 (1.73–2.81)	.0855
Suicidal plans	3.05 (2.46–3.79)	2.71 (2.19–3.36)	2.24 (1.76–2.85)	3.15 (2.33–4.25)	2.53 (1.93–3.33)	.3745
Suicide attempts	3.46 (2.55–4.68)	4.03 (2.90–5.60)	3.12 (2.33–4.17)	3.98 (2.84–5.56)	2.66 (1.97–3.61)	.3401
Suicide injury	3.73 (2.15–6.47)	4.43 (2.99–6.55)	5.35 (3.23–8.87)	3.21 (1.88–5.50)	4.75 (2.50–9.06)	.8007
Both online and offline victimization (reference: none)						
Suicidal ideation	5.30 (4.34–6.46)	6.35 (5.48–7.35)	6.78 (5.63–8.15)	5.84 (4.92–6.94)	5.00 (4.23–5.91)	.0845
Suicidal plans	5.24 (4.18–6.57)	5.58 (4.68–6.65)	6.25 (4.95–7.89)	5.11 (4.17–6.27)	4.88 (4.11–5.79)	.5222
Suicide attempts	5.66 (4.55–7.03)	7.31 (5.82–9.17)	7.92 (6.01–10.43)	7.28 (5.67–9.36)	5.91 (4.64–7.52)	.2915
Suicide injury	4.33 (2.77–6.76)	10.49 (7.22–15.25)	11.33 (8.16–15.72)	8.90 (6.34–12.50)	7.66 (5.08–11.55)	.0149

Adjusted for race and ethnicity and sex.

Still, the strong risk for suicidal ideation, plans, attempts and injury that accompanies both online and offline peer victimization remains a powerful determinant of adolescent health. This is especially true for students being bullied both online and offline who not only faced substantially higher odds of suicidal outcomes compared with those who were not bullied but typically had approximately twice the odds of any given outcome compared with those who were bullied either online only or offline only. Although victimization did not explain the trends in suicidal outcomes, the harmful psychosocial impact of peer victimization cannot be overstated. Our results align with similar findings linking offline and online victimization to suicidal outcomes,[19-22] including studies that use smaller subsets of YRBS data,[23-25] and suicidal symptom outcomes are just some of the adverse mental health consequences of being victimized, along with depression,[26,27] anxiety,[21] and low self-esteem.[28,29] These psychological factors, together with loneliness and hopelessness, have been hypothesized as possible mediators linking victimization to suicidal outcomes, although the causal structure of these connections is still being explored.[30-33]

Reducing peer victimization remains a challenging and important goal, particularly as prevalence is remaining flat despite substantial national investment in efforts to reduce peer victimization and bullying. Literature supporting these efforts suggests that programs that are sustained longer are more effective,[34] as opposed to single assemblies for bullying awareness.[35] Empirically supported components, such as parental engagement and education,[36] consistent administrative monitoring and enforcement of programs,[36] and bystander training for students[37] may be underutilized.

However, there is growing evidence that these programs may not be effective for older adolescents,[38] given the shift to more relational (eg, rumors) rather than direct (eg, hitting) forms of victimization and the dynamic nature of social interaction among older adolescents. Intervention effectiveness studies should isolate samples of older adolescents and tailor programs to this population. Additionally, the long-term impact of certain interventions may have unintended consequences of harming certain adolescents, even if the overall environment is healthier.[39] This is known as the healthy context paradox and may stem from added self-blame, isolation, or targeting of specific adolescents by bullies as fewer peers face victimization. Reinforcing messaging and norms that reduce victim blame for violence and feelings of isolation (ie, sharing that others have faced similar hardships) while

TABLE 4 aORs for Suicide Outcomes Based on Experiences of Victimization by Year, Female, 2011–2019 YRBS

Victimization Experience Predictor, Suicidal Behavior Outcome	2011, aOR (95% CI)	2013, aOR (95% CI)	2015, aOR (95% CI)	2017, aOR (95% CI)	2019, aOR (95% CI)	*P* for Interaction Between Year and Victimization
Offline victimization (reference: none)						
Suicidal ideation	2.76 (2.13–3.58)	2.98 (2.38–3.72)	3.02 (2.54–3.59)	2.95 (2.35–3.72)	2.54 (2.07–3.11)	.7923
Suicidal plans	2.81 (2.25–3.52)	2.82 (2.23–3.57)	2.69 (2.12–3.43)	3.00 (2.30–3.92)	2.70 (2.18–3.35)	.9824
Suicide attempts	2.17 (1.63–2.91)	3.09 (2.34–4.09)	2.63 (1.86–3.72)	3.88 (2.90–5.19)	2.62 (1.96–3.49)	.1160
Suicide injury	1.82 (0.77–4.33)	3.00 (2.01–4.48)	2.80 (1.66–4.73)	3.96 (2.28–6.88)	1.80 (0.93–3.51)	.4202
Online victimization (reference: none)						
Suicidal ideation	3.34 (2.58–4.32)	2.84 (2.25–3.59)	2.79 (2.23–3.49)	2.79 (2.07–3.77)	2.07 (1.55–2.76)	.2742
Suicidal plans	2.78 (2.15–3.61)	2.63 (2.08–3.33)	2.04 (1.63–2.54)	2.79 (1.90–4.12)	2.45 (1.81–3.32)	.3972
Suicide attempts	2.88 (1.99–4.18)	3.45 (2.48–4.81)	2.54 (1.88–3.42)	3.83 (2.48–5.90)	2.37 (1.64–3.41)	.3755
Suicide injury	3.21 (1.60–6.42)	3.67 (2.29–5.90)	3.76 (2.30–6.14)	3.36 (1.70–6.61)	3.44 (1.71–6.93)	.9939
Both online and offline victimization (reference: none)						
Suicidal ideation	5.39 (4.27–6.80)	5.97 (4.78–7.45)	7.03 (5.54–8.91)	5.55 (4.49–6.86)	4.64 (3.79–5.69)	.1408
Suicidal plans	5.20 (4.12–6.55)	5.27 (4.18–6.64)	5.70 (4.28–7.59)	5.07 (4.03–6.38)	4.54 (3.72–5.54)	.7655
Suicide attempts	5.15 (4.02–6.60)	6.95 (5.23–9.24)	7.16 (5.18–9.90)	7.40 (5.68–9.63)	5.69 (4.36–7.43)	.3226
Suicide injury	4.91 (3.01–8.01)	8.62 (5.71–13.00)	9.39 (6.09–14.47)	7.77 (5.36–11.28)	7.03 (4.18–11.83)	.3723

Adjusted for race and ethnicity.

empowering victims to seek help is crucial. Current violence reduction programs are likely insufficient, as evidenced by the stagnant trends in victimization.

Fundamentally, our findings indicate that the patterns of victimization seem to be changing, with many young people being victimized both online and offline, and so interventions must be designed and evaluated to address this co-occurring victimization. With offline victimization, the threat of physical violence exists and so a programmatic emphasis on teaching and enforcing nonviolence is warranted. Progress achieved for more traditional forms of victimization may be offset by new forms of victimization, especially as new digital social platforms provide novel spaces and methods for peer victimization. With online victimization, harm may be more direct without any possibility of intervention from bystanders. Perpetrators may find it easier to bully given the distance and potential anonymity of online harassment, leading to more enduring or persistent victimization. School administrations and parents maintaining open communication about safety online and monitoring issues as they arise are just some potential ways to recognize and handle this problem.

Although connections between victimization and suicidal outcomes are etiologically important for prevention, they do not explain the recent increases in suicidal ideation or plans given that victimization has not increased in the United States. Explanation for suicidal trends, therefore, should focus on other areas. Risk factors such as sleep quality and duration[40–43] as well as mood symptoms and affective disorders[44] are promising explanatory mechanisms for the increase in suicidal outcomes given trends that coincide with the increase in suicidal ideation and plans.

Limitations

For individual adolescents, the cross-sectional nature of the YRBS does not permit temporal ordering of victimization and suicidal outcomes, preventing causal attribution. Although the hypothesized association is that peer victimization leads to worsened mental health and increased suicidal outcomes, the reverse is plausible, wherein adolescents who are struggling emotionally may face more victimization or may perceive peer interactions as more hostile. These represent different pathways that longitudinal data can disentangle, although both may operate simultaneously.

Suicide items were limited. For suicidal ideation, students only report whether these thoughts are present, not their frequency or intensity. Similarly, victimization in both forms was self-reported as having occurred or not, rather than the frequency or content of the

TABLE 5 aORs for Suicide Outcomes Based on Experiences of Victimization by Year, Male, 2011–2019 YRBS

Victimization Experience Predictor, Suicidal Behavior Outcome	2011, aOR (95% CI)	2013, aOR (95% CI)	2015, aOR (95% CI)	2017, aOR (95% CI)	2019, aOR (95% CI)	*P* for Interaction Between Year and Victimization
Offline victimization (reference: none)						
Suicidal ideation	2.52 (1.92–3.31)	2.69 (2.00–3.63)	2.81 (2.17–3.64)	3.36 (2.58–4.37)	2.82 (2.01–3.94)	.5730
Suicidal plans	2.58 (1.83–3.65)	2.58 (1.93–3.43)	1.92 (1.47–2.50)	3.62 (2.77–4.73)	3.01 (2.11–4.29)	.0225
Suicide attempts	2.55 (1.73–3.77)	2.39 (1.53–3.74)	3.13 (1.98–4.96)	3.21 (2.01–5,14)	2.62 (1.61–4.27)	.8827
Suicide injury	1.52 (0.78–2.89)	2.55 (1.27–5.11)	3.67 (1.84–7.31)	4.47 (2.18–9.18)	3.34 (1.38–8.09)	.2516
Online victimization (reference: none)						
Suicidal ideation	3.20 (2.24–4.58)	2.89 (1.69–4.97)	2.15 (1.33–3.45)	5.17 (3.46–7.71)	2.49 (1.52–4.08)	.0431
Suicidal plans	3.69 (2.58–5.27)	2.92 (1.90–4.48)	2.82 (1.65–4.82)	4.03 (2.72–5.96)	2.70 (1.47–4.93)	.2677
Suicide attempts	5.04 (3.16–8.02)	5.76 (3.14–10.59)	4.84 (2.53–9.26)	4.50 (2.42–8.35)	3.45 (1.81–6.56)	.8024
Suicide injury	5.17 (2.64–10.13)	6.04 (3.04–12.01)	9.87 (3.58–27.24)	2.26 (0.79–6.44)	8.67 (3.21–23.45)	.4360
Both online and offline victimization (reference: none)						
Suicidal ideation	5.35 (3.95–7.25)	7.87 (5.80–10.66)	6.44 (5.20–7.97)	6.69 (4.94–9.05)	5.84 (4.34–7.86)	.5412
Suicidal plans	5.50 (3.45–8.76)	6.69 (4.80–9.32)	7.79 (5.67–10.71)	5.37 (3.83–7.53)	5.77 (4.33–7.69)	.6393
Suicide attempts	6.68 (4.78–9.32)	8.31 (5.89–11.71)	9.82 (6.22–15.52)	7.50 (4.54–12.40)	6.54 (4.25–10.08)	.7819
Suicide injury	3.10 (1.54–6.24)	15.14 (9.11–25.16)	15.23 (8.58–27.03)	12.82 (6.61–24.89)	8.36 (4.22–16.55)	.0040

Adjusted for race and ethnicity.

victimization. Offline victimization only dealt with instances on school property, so victimization not on school grounds could not be captured. Lastly, other potentially important covariates, like mental health diagnosis and socioeconomic status, were not available in these data, and so their exclusion from models, while unavoidable, is a limitation of these models.

Certain YRBS years lack data from individual states, limiting the extent to which data are nationally representative. For instance, in 2019, Oregon, Washington, Wyoming, and Minnesota did not participate.[13] These data also do not represent students outside of the school systems where surveying occurs and so do not capture homeschooled students or homeless youth not attending school.

Conclusions

Although experiences of victimization predict suicidal ideation, plans, attempts and injury, victimization trends do not explain the worrying increases seen in suicidal ideation and plans. Victimization prevention efforts should be strengthened with the acknowledgment that victimization, both online and offline, is a major risk factor for adolescent suicidal outcomes, especially when these forms of victimization co-occur. To explain the recent increases in suicidal ideation and plans, researchers must look beyond victimization.

ABBREVIATIONS

aOR: adjusted odds ratio
CI: confidence interval
OR: odds ratio
YRBS: Youth Risk Behavior Survey

PEDIATRICS (ISSN Numbers: Print, 0031-4005; Online, 1098-4275).

Address correspondence to Noah Kreski, Department of Epidemiology, Columbia University, Mailman School of Public Health, New York, New York. E-mail: ntk2109@columbia.edu

PEDIATRICS (ISSN Numbers: Print, 0031-4005; Online, 1098-4275).

FINANCIAL DISCLOSURE: The authors have indicated they have no financial relationships relevant to this article to disclose.

FUNDING: Funded by grant R01DA048853 (PI: Keyes) and with support from the Columbia Center for Injury Science and Prevention (R49-CE003094). Additionally, Dr Martins reports funding from grant R01DA037866, Dr Hasin reports funding from grant R01DA048860, and Dr Mauro reports funding from grant K01DA045224. The funder had no role in the design and conduct of the study. Funded by the National Institutes of Health (NIH).

POTENTIAL CONFLICT OF INTEREST: The authors have indicated they have no conflicts of interest to disclose.

REFERENCES

1. Centers for Disease Control and Prevention, National Center for Injury Prevention and Control. *Web-based Injury Statistics Query and Reporting System (WISQARS)* [online]. 2005. Available at: www.cdc.gov/injury/wisqars. Accessed July 13, 2021
2. Burstein B, Agostino H, Greenfield B. Suicidal attempts and ideation among children and adolescents in us emergency departments, 2007-2015. *JAMA Pediatr.* 2019;173(6):598–600
3. Pontes NMH, Ayres CG, Pontes MCF. Trends in depressive symptoms and suicidality: youth risk behavior survey 2009-2017. *Nurs Res.* 2020;69(3):176–185
4. Kann L, McManus T, Harris WA, et al. Youth risk behavior surveillance - United States, 2017. *MMWR Surveill Summ.* 2018;67(8):1–114
5. Centers for Disease Control and Prevention. *Trends in the Prevalence of Suicide-Related Behaviors National YRBS: 1991-2017.* Atlanta, GA: Centers for Disease Control and Prevention; 2017
6. Bannink R, Broeren S, van de Looij-Jansen PM, de Waart FG, Raat H. Cyber and traditional bullying victimization as a risk factor for mental health problems and suicidal ideation in adolescents. *PLoS One.* 2014;9(4):e94026
7. Hinduja S, Patchin JW.. Connecting adolescent suicide to the severity of bullying and cyberbullying. *J Sch Violence.* 2019;18(3):333–346
8. Koyanagi A, Oh H, Carvalho AF, et al. Bullying victimization and suicide attempt among adolescents aged 12-15 years from 48 countries. *J Am Acad Child Adolesc Psychiatry.* 2019;58(9):907–918.e4
9. John A, Glendenning AC, Marchant A, et al. Self-harm, suicidal behaviours, and cyberbullying in children and young people: systematic review. *J Med Internet Res.* 2018;20(4):e129
10. Gunn JF III, Goldstein SE. Bullying and suicidal behavior during adolescence: a developmental perspective. *Adolesc Res Rev.* 2017;2:77–97
11. Kowalski RM, Morgan CA, Limber SP. Traditional bullying as a potential warning sign of cyberbullying. *Sch Psychol Int.* 2012;33(5):505–519
12. Modecki KL, Minchin J, Harbaugh AG, Guerra NG, Runions KC. Bullying prevalence across contexts: A meta-analysis measuring cyber and traditional bullying. *J Adolesc Health.* 2014;55(5):602–611
13. Underwood JM, Brener N, Thornton J, et al. Overview and methods for the youth risk behavior surveillance system - United States. 2019. *MMWR Suppl.* 2020;69(1):1–10
14. May A, Klonsky ED. Validity of suicidality items from the Youth Risk Behavior Survey in a high school sample. *Assessment.* 2011;18(3):379–381
15. Xu M, Macrynikola N, Waseem M, Miranda R. Racial and ethnic differences in bullying: Review and implications for intervention. *Aggress Violent Behav.* 2020;50:101340
16. Lee CS, Wong YJ. Racial/ethnic and gender differences in the antecedents of youth suicide. *Cultur Divers Ethnic Minor Psychol.* 2020;26(4):532–543
17. Ivey-Stephenson AZ, Demissie Z, Crosby AE, et al. Suicidal ideation and behaviors among high school students - Youth Risk Behavior Survey, United States, 2019. *MMWR Suppl.* 2020;69(1):47–55
18. Li R, Lian Q, Su Q, Li L, Xie M, Hu J. Trends and sex disparities in school bullying victimization among U.S. youth, 2011-2019. *BMC Public Health.* 2020;20(1):1583
19. Hinduja S, Patchin JW. Bullying, cyberbullying, and suicide. *Arch Suicide Res.* 2010;14(3):206–221
20. Brunstein Klomek A, Sourander A, Gould M. The association of suicide and bullying in childhood to young adulthood: a review of cross-sectional and longitudinal research findings. *Can J Psychiatry.* 2010;55(5):282–288
21. Moore SE, Norman RE, Suetani S, Thomas HJ, Sly PD, Scott JG. Consequences of bullying victimization in childhood and adolescence: a systematic review and meta-analysis. *World J Psychiatry.* 2017;7(1):60–76
22. van Geel M, Vedder P, Tanilon J. Relationship between peer victimization, cyberbullying, and suicide in children and adolescents: a meta-analysis. *JAMA Pediatr.* 2014;168(5):435–442
23. Messias E, Kindrick K, Castro J. School bullying, cyberbullying, or both: correlates of teen suicidality in the 2011 CDC Youth Risk Behavior Survey. *Compr Psychiatry.* 2014;55(5):1063–1068
24. Reed KP, Nugent W, Cooper RL. Testing a path model of relationships between gender, age, and bullying victimization and violent behavior, substance abuse, depression, suicidal ideation, and suicide attempts in adolescents. *Child Youth Serv Rev.* 2015;55:128–137
25. Alhajji M, Bass S, Dai T. Cyberbullying, mental health, and violence in adolescents and associations with sex and race: data from the 2015 Youth Risk Behavior Survey. *Glob Pediatr Heal.* 2019;6:2333794X19868887
26. Brunstein Klomek A, Marrocco F, Kleinman M, Schonfeld IS, Gould MS. Bullying, depression, and suicidality in adolescents. *J Am Acad Child Adolesc Psychiatry.* 2007;46(1):40–49
27. Arseneault L, Bowes L, Shakoor S. Bullying victimization in youths and mental health problems: 'much ado about nothing'? *Psychol Med.* 2010;40(5):717–729
28. van Geel M, Goemans A, Zwaanswijk W, Gini G, Vedder P. Does peer victimization predict low self-esteem, or does low self-esteem predict peer victimization? Meta-analyses on longitudinal studies. *Dev Rev.* 2018;49:31–40
29. Tsaousis I. The relationship of self-esteem to bullying perpetration and peer victimization among schoolchildren and adolescents: a meta-analytic review. *Aggress Violent Behav.* 2016;31:186–199

30. Hong JS, Kral MJ, Sterzing PR. Pathways from bullying perpetration, victimization, and bully victimization to suicidality among school-aged youth: a review of the potential mediators and a call for further investigation. trauma, violence. *Trauma Violence Abuse*. 2015;16(4):379–390

31. Bauman S, Toomey RB, Walker JL. Associations among bullying, cyberbullying, and suicide in high school students. *J Adolesc*. 2013;36(2):341–350

32. Sampasa-Kanyinga H, Roumeliotis P, Xu H. Associations between cyberbullying and school bullying victimization and suicidal ideation, plans and attempts among Canadian schoolchildren. *PLoS One*. 2014;9(7):e102145

33. Bonanno RA, Hymel S. Beyond hurt feelings investigating why some victims of bullying are at greater risk for suicidal ideation. *Merrill-Palmer Q*. 2010;56(3):420–440

34. Fox BH, Farrington DP, Ttofi MM. Successful bullying prevention programs: influence of research design, implementation features, and program components. *Int J Conf Violence*. 2012;6(2):273–283

35. Bradshaw CP. Translating research to practice in bullying prevention. *Am Psychol*. 2015;70(4):322–332

36. Gaffney H, Ttofi MM, Farrington DP. Evaluating the effectiveness of school-bullying prevention programs: an updated meta-analytical review. *Aggress Violent Behav*. 2019;45:111–133

37. Nickerson AB, Aloe AM, Livingston JA, Feeley TH. Measurement of the bystander intervention model for bullying and sexual harassment. *J Adolesc*. 2014;37(4):391–400

38. Yeager DS, Fong CJ, Lee HY, Espelage DL. Declines in efficacy of anti-bullying programs among older adolescents: theory and a three-level meta-analysis. *J Appl Dev Psychol*. 2015;37:36–51

39. Healy KL. Hypotheses for possible iatrogenic impacts of school bullying prevention programs. *Child Dev Perspect*. 2020;14(4):221–228

40. Liu X, Liu ZZ, Wang ZY, Yang Y, Liu BP, Jia CX. Daytime sleepiness predicts future suicidal behavior: a longitudinal study of adolescents. *Sleep (Basel)*. 2019;42(2):

41. Wong MM, Brower KJ. The prospective relationship between sleep problems and suicidal behavior in the National Longitudinal Study of Adolescent Health. *J Psychiatr Res*. 2012;46(7):953–959

42. Mars B, Heron J, Klonsky ED, et al. Predictors of future suicide attempt among adolescents with suicidal thoughts or non-suicidal self-harm: a population-based birth cohort study. *Lancet Psychiatry*. 2019;6(4):327–337

43. Chiu HY, Lee HC, Chen PY, Lai YF, Tu YK. Associations between sleep duration and suicidality in adolescents: A systematic review and dose-response meta-analysis. *Sleep Med Rev*. 2018;42:119–126

44. Gili M, Castellví P, Vives M, et al. Mental disorders as risk factors for suicidal behavior in young people: A meta-analysis and systematic review of longitudinal studies. *J Affect Disord*. 2019; 245:152–162

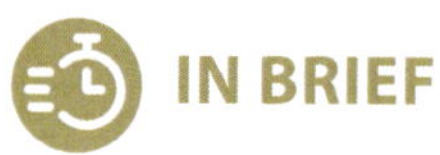

#TechAddicted: Understanding Problematic Internet Use in Adolescents

Anna F. Jolliff, MS,* Megan A. Moreno, MD, MSEd, MPH*

*Department of Pediatrics, University of Wisconsin, Madison, WI

With the increasing availability and use of digital and electronic media, researchers have increasingly focused on quantifying its healthy and unhealthy uses. From this effort have emerged tools to define and detect problematic use of media and technology. The vast majority of this research and related tools pertain specifically to media that are connected to the Internet, such as online gambling, Internet gaming, and social media. Problematic Internet use (PIU) has become an important public health issue among adolescents, and thus it is relevant to pediatricians.

Early work and definitions of electronic addiction focused on the concept of Internet addiction. Definitions of Internet addiction were directly translated from the diagnostic criteria associated with other types of addiction, such as alcohol use disorder. Most models of Internet addiction include symptoms associated with substance misuse, such as using the Internet to regulate one's mood or loss of control while using the Internet. Somewhat lacking from this framework, however, has been an acknowledgment that use of the Internet can be problematic and clinically significant in the absence of outcomes or features traditionally associated with addiction to chemical substances.

In the past decade, PIU has emerged as the preferred construct in the literature and in clinical settings. In contrast to the narrow focus of Internet addiction, PIU has been defined as "internet use that is risky, excessive or impulsive in nature, leading to adverse life consequences, specifically physical, emotional, social, or functional impairment." (Moreno et al., 2013) In a clinical setting, use of the construct PIU has at least two major benefits. First, it acknowledges that impairment or negative life consequences may result from the problematic use of media without otherwise resembling addiction as it is traditionally conceptualized. And second, the measurement tool associated with PIU, the Problematic and Risky Internet Use Screening Scale (PRIUSS), is not specific to one electronic medium, giving it broader clinical utility and relevance over time. The PRIUSS can detect PIU overall and can also detect problematic use of subtypes of electronic media, such as video games, social media, gambling, and the use of smartphones. Furthermore, the PRIUSS remains the only validated English language screening tool with a robust evidence base in the scientific literature.

Prevalence estimates for PIU vary by population. With the PRIUSS as a measurement tool, prevalence has ranged from 9% to 11% in college samples in the United States. Subsets of PIU have shown somewhat different prevalence rates. For example, Internet gaming disorder has shown rates of 1.16% in German adolescents and 10.8% in Korean adolescents. Social media addiction (as measured by the Bergen Social Media Addiction Scale) showed a prevalence of 4.5% among Hungarian

AUTHOR DISCLOSURE Ms Jolliff and Dr Moreno have disclosed no financial relationships relevant to this article. This commentary does not contain a discussion of an unapproved/investigative use of a commercial product/device.

SUGGESTED READINGS

Problematic Internet Use among US Youth: A Systematic Review. Moreno MA, Jelenchick L, Cox E, Young H, Christakis DA. *Arch Pediatr Adolesc Med.* 2011;165(9):797–805

Problematic Internet Use among Older Adolescents: A Conceptual Framework. Moreno MA, Jelenchick LA, Christakis DA. *Comput Human Behav.* 2013;29(4), 1879–1887

The Problematic and Risky Internet Use Screening Scale (PRIUSS) for Adolescents and Young Adults: Scale Development and Refinement. Jelenchick LA, Eickhoff J, Christakis DA, et al. *Comput Human Behav.* 2014;35:10.1016/j.chb.2014.01.035

Media Use in School-Aged Children and Adolescents. Council on Communications and Media. *Pediatrics.* 2016;138(5):e20162592

adolescents. Measurement of PIU is complicated by research showing that people may not accurately report their own Internet use.

Despite the challenges in reporting, assessing, and understanding PIU, efforts have been made to articulate (and, ultimately, prevent) its development in the individual. Why is it that in today's digitally immersed society, some people develop PIU and others do not? As with other mental health disorders, the answer must account for dispositional and environmental factors. At least two primary environmental mechanisms have been posited. One suggests that Internet use that is in its nature excessive leads to the development of PIU, regardless of the specific activities performed online. Another suggests that particular types of Internet use (eg, viewing pornography or engaging with social media) promote addiction, because these activities may trigger the release of dopamine or are otherwise particularly rewarding. Similar to the development of other behavioral addictions, much work remains to be done before the genesis or mechanisms of PIU are understood.

Just as the process of development is an outstanding question, so is the question of who is most at risk. Studies are conflicting in this area. Some suggest that females are more at risk for PIU, and others suggest that the same is true for men and older teens. PIU is more common in people with other comorbid mental and physical health conditions, including attention-deficit/hyperactivity disorder, depression, and social anxiety, as well as sleep difficulties, reduced physical activity, and less healthy eating. Research suggests that socioeconomic status is also associated with PIU; it may be that for adolescents in less privileged homes, parents are not available to actively monitor the media use of their children.

Treatment for electronic addiction resembles treatment for other behavioral addictions and may include extended periods of time without the medium and development of new, healthier replacement behaviors. Unfortunately, no evidence-based treatment approaches for PIU are currently available in the United States. Given the difficulty and cost associated with treating any behavioral addiction, prevention is paramount and starts at home. Parents should be encouraged to model the appropriate use of media for their children as well as to set explicit boundaries around media engagement. The American Academy of Pediatrics (AAP) has put forth guidelines on media use, which include limiting both the amount of screen media use and the types of media used, as well as encouraging families to identify media-free times and locations in the home:

1. For children younger than 18 months, avoid screen media (other than video-chatting).
2. Limit screen use to 1 hour per day of high-quality viewing for children 2 to 5 years old.
3. For older children and adolescents, put consistent limits on the time and types of media use, making sure it does not interfere with adequate sleep, physical activity, and other age-appropriate healthy behaviors. Designate media-free times (dinner and driving) and media-free areas (bedrooms). Have ongoing conversations about online safety and treating everyone with respect.

The past decade has seen enormous strides in defining and understanding PIU, particularly in conceptualizing PIU as a broader, more clinically relevant concept compared with Internet addiction. Significant areas of need for future research include appropriate prevention and intervention strategies. Two key tools available for clinicians include 1) the PRIUSS for use in primary care settings and 2) the Family Media Use Plan, a tool derived from the AAP's 2016 media use guidelines. This tool can empower families to define and develop personalized strategies for healthy media use at home.

COMMENT: Prevention is, of course, far preferable to treatment. The AAP 2016 Guidelines on Media Use emphasize the role parents must play in supervising their children's engagement with electronic media, both in setting limits and in actively encouraging conversations that can lead to mutual understanding. But experience should warn us that powerful forces beyond the family's reach are involved. The tech companies behind social media, Internet gaming, online gambling, and the such have a vested interest in promoting the use of their products, as did tobacco companies and, more recently, the vaping industry. Profits are the bottom line. Product design as well as advertising are designed to attract customers, and children and adolescents are an attractive and lucrative target. Once again, we need active advocacy by the pediatric community, individually as well as through the AAP, in pushing for regulation of the ever-expanding tech world now seemingly omnipresent, but hopefully not yet omnipotent.

–Henry M. Adam, MD
Associate Editor, *In Brief*

Screens for Calming: Use Caution

Source: *Radesky JS, Kaciroti N, Weeks HM, et al. Longitudinal associations between use of mobile devices for calming and emotional reactivity and executive functioning in children aged 3 to 5 years [published online ahead of print December 12, 2022]. JAMA Pediatr. doi:10.1001/jamapediatrics.2022.4793*

Investigators from the University of Michigan, Ann Arbor, MI, conducted a longitudinal cohort study to assess the bidirectional associations between use of mobile devices for calming and executive functioning (EF) and emotional reactivity in young children. Study participants were typically developing children 3 to 5 years old whose parents owned at least 1 mobile device. Study data were collected using web-based surveys completed by the parents of enrolled children, with surveys including demographic information, use of mobile devices for calming, measures of EF and emotional reactivity, and child temperament. The use of mobile devices for calming was measured at baseline (T1), at 3 months (T2), and at 6 months (T3) by asking parents to rate how likely they were to give their child a mobile device to use when they were upset. Possible responses ranged from 0 (not at all likely) to 4 (very likely). EF was assessed at T1, T2, and T3 using the Behavior Rating Inventory of Executive Function-Preschool version, with higher scores indicative of reduced EF. Emotional reactivity also was assessed at all time points using the emotional reactivity subscale on the Child Behavior Checklist-Preschool, with higher scores indicative of more reactivity. Finally, child surgent temperament was assessed using the surgency subscale on the Rothbart Child Behavior Questionnaire-Very Short form; scores were dichotomized to categorize study participants has high or low surgency. Path model analyses assessed cross-lagged (exposure at T1 with outcome at T2, or exposure at T2 with outcome at T3) bidirectional correlations between use of mobile devices for calming and EF or emotional reactivity. Four sets of analyses were conducted, stratified on sex and high and low surgency, after adjusting for multiple demographic characteristics.

A total of 422 children with a mean age of 3.8 ±0.5 years were enrolled. At T1, 8.5% of parents reported being very likely to use mobile devices to calm their child when upset. Among boy participants, use of device calming at T2 was significantly associated with emotional reactivity at T3 ($r = 0.20$; 95% CI, 0.10, 0.30), but emotional reactivity at T2 was not statistically associated with use of device calming at T3. In girls, use of device calming at T1 was associated with EF at T2 ($r = 0.12$; 95% CI, 0.03, 0.22). Among participants with high surgency, device calming at T2 was significantly associated with emotional reactivity at T3, and emotional reactivity at T2 was associated with use of calming devices at T3 ($r = 0.11$; 95% CI, 0.01, 0.22, and $r = 0.13$; 95% CI, 0.02, 0.24, respectively). There were no statistically significant crossed-lagged associations between use of device calming and either EF or emotional reactivity in children with low surgency.

The authors conclude that frequent use of mobile devices for calming young children may affect their emotional reactivity.

COMMENTARY BY

Mike Dubik, MD, FAAP, Pediatrics and Sleep Medicine, Naval Medical Center Portsmouth, Portsmouth, VA

Dr Dubik has disclosed no financial relationship relevant to this commentary. This commentary does not contain a discussion of an unapproved/investigative use of a commercial product/device.

Mobile devices are often used to keep young children occupied or calm.[1] Is the use of mobile device screen time to calm a toddler negatively associated with their development of executive functions and emotional regulation? The results of the current study confirm others that have found that screen viewing in the wrong context impairs the development of executive functions and school readiness.[2,3]

The AAP recommends that young children not use media more than 1 hour per day and that media should be high-quality and co-viewed, as part of a Family Media Use Plan.[4] Yet researchers in 2017 reported that children under 5 years of age averaged 2.4 hours per day of screen time. And, of course, media use increased during the COVID-19 pandemic.[5]

Parents can find themselves in difficult situations.[6] Mobile devices can distract or assuage but if used habitually can hamper emotional development.

Limitations of the current study included the use of a single question to assess the use of mobile devices for calming purposes and enrolling participants through the use of a community-based convenience sample.

The results of this prospective cohort study support the AAP recommendation for the limited and judicious use of media to calm an infant or toddler.[4] The results also confirm the wording of an earlier AAP recommendation: "Unstructured playtime is more valuable for the developing brain than any electronic media exposure."[7] The authors suggest that the frequent use of mobile devices for calming young children be avoided.

Bottom Line: An over-reliance on mobile devices to calm a toddler may adversely affect development of executive functions and emotional regulation.

References

1. Radesky JS, et al. *Pediatrics.* 2020;146(1):e20193518; doi: 10.1542/peds.2019-3518.
2. McHarg G, et al. *Front Psychol.* 2020;11:570392; doi: 10.3389/fpsyg.2020.570392.
3. Lawrence A, Choe DE. *Acad Pediatr.* 2021;21(6);996-1000; doi: 10.1016/j.acap.2021.01.007.
4. Radesky J, Council on Communications and Media, et al. *Pediatrics.* 2016;138(5):e20162591; doi: 10.1542/peds.2016-2591.
5. Shutzman B, Gershy N. *Comput Human Behav.* 2023;139:107559; doi: 10.1016/j.chb.2022.107559
6. Mallawaarachchi SR, et al. *BMC Public Health.* 2022;22(1):2011; doi: 10.1186/s12889-022-14459-0.
7. Brown A, Council on Communications and Media. *Pediatrics.* 2011;128(5):1040-1045; doi: 10.1542/peds.2011-1753.

RESEARCH ARTICLE

A Quality Improvement Initiative to Reduce Screen Time in a Children's Hospital

Anna Schmitz, MD, Heather Eastman, BSN, Robin Ostegaard, CCLS and Stephanie Stewart, PhD

ABSTRACT

OBJECTIVES: The American Academy of Pediatrics strongly recommends that children age 2 and under should have little to no digital media exposure. However, most children are exposed to regular screen time at home. This may also be true for hospitalized children. Through education and access to alternatives, we aimed to reduce screen exposure in our children's hospital for children 2 and under.

METHODS: Between January 2020 and May 2021, we designed and implemented a quality improvement intervention to educate staff and caregivers on the American Academy of Pediatrics screen time recommendations and offer alternatives for hospitalized children. Our primary aim was to decrease screen time exposure for children age 2 and under by 50% within 12 months of project initiation. Balancing measures included staff perception of workload when using screens and perceived parental acceptance of screens being turned off.

RESULTS: During baseline data collection period, screens were on for an average of 63% of the audits. Following interventions, the average was reduced to 40%. The outcome measure met special cause with 8 consecutive points below the center line. There was a significant increase in staff who reported offering screen alternatives after intervention. Staff perception of workload and perceived parental acceptance was unchanged.

CONCLUSIONS: Through implementation of this quality improvement initiative, we reduced screen time by approximately 37% without impacting staff workload. Most importantly, we were able to educate staff and model best practices for caregivers, which may carry into the home, leading to a reduction of screen time and improved health overall.

www.hospitalpediatrics.org
DOI:https://doi.org/10.1542/hpeds.2021-006236

Address correspondence to Anna Schmitz, MD, Department of Pediatrics, Stead Family Children's Hospital, 200 Hawkins Dr. BT1333, Iowa City, IA 52242. E-mail: anna-schmitz@uiowa.edu

University of Iowa Stead Family Children's Hospital, Iowa City, Iowa

HOSPITAL PEDIATRICS (ISSN Numbers: Print, 2154-1663; Online, 2154-1671).

FUNDING: No external funding.

CONFLICT OF INTEREST DISCLOSURES: The authors have indicated they have no conflicts of interest to disclose.

Dr Schmitz conceptualized and designed the study, designed the data collection instruments, collected data, conducted the initial analyses, drafted the initial manuscript, and reviewed and revised the manuscript; Ms Stewart, Ms Eastman, and Ms Ostegaard contributed to study design, including the data collection instruments and reviewed and revised the manuscript; and all authors approved the final manuscript as submitted and agree to be accountable for all aspects of the work.

The American Academy of Pediatrics (AAP) has made a strong recommendation that children age 2 and under should have little to no digital media exposure.[1] Regular exposure to screen media may interfere with language and cognitive development, in addition to sleep quality.[2,3] The extent of this interference depends on the program content and amount of exposure to screen time.[1–3] Specifically, for children age 2 and under, there are negative associations with language and executive function development.[3] Screen media exposure in the evening has been linked with shorter sleep duration and fewer minutes of sleep for children, including infants.[1] For older children and adolescents, there are other negative impacts of excessive digital media use, including obesity, poor sleep, attention problems, and impaired social coping.[4]

The AAP recommends for infants and toddlers less than age 2, unless used for live video chat, screen time should be minimized as much as possible. For children aged 2 to 5, the AAP recommends up to 2 hours per day of educational programming.[1] Ideally caregivers should co-view to enhance understanding of high-quality program content. Most children are exposed to excessive screen time at home. Parents report that children watch more than 2 hours per day of television (TV), not including tablet and smart phone use.[5] A cross-sectional study in a low-income, minority community showed nearly universal mobile device use among children less than 4 years old.[6] They found by age 2, most children were using these devices daily and by age 4, 75% of the children had their own device.[6]

Hospitalized children are at risk for excessive screen exposure.[7,8] Survey results published by Arora et al revealed almost half of caregivers felt the amount of screen media used by their child when hospitalized was more than they would like.[7] This study showed that digital media use was noted in over half (59.9%) of observations of hospitalized children less than 2 years old. Another hospital reported in an observational study that 91% of all pediatric inpatients had the TV turned on.[6] The AAP guidelines outline inappropriate content for young children as programs rated PG-13, R, and PG or G programs centered on adult themes. Using this system, they found that children 2 years and younger had the highest exposure to inappropriate content at 74% and higher when an adult is present.[8]

Hospitals have been quick to implement digital screens in patient rooms, but slow to educate patients and caregivers on ideal utilization and risks of excessive exposure. Pediatricians frequently serve as liaison for caregivers and are responsible for endorsing AAP recommendations. Hospitalization provides frequent and direct communication between staff and caregivers, creating an opportune time for education. Therefore, we included education and modeling as we conducted a quality improvement initiative (QI) to decrease digital screen exposure by 50% over a 12-month period for inpatient children 2 years of age and younger.

METHODS

Project Setting and Participants

An interdisciplinary team led by a pediatric hospitalist at a midwestern, academic children's hospital designed a QI initiative for inpatient children age 2 and under. Our institutional review board determined this study to not be human subject's research. Our children's hospital is a tertiary-care academic children's hospital with 190 beds housed in a building opened in 2017 with state-of-the-art technology designed to enhance the overall experience. In each inpatient room, children and caregivers have access to an interactive system consisting of a TV screen and a bedside tablet.

The focus of this project was on children age 2 and under admitted to an acute care pediatric floor of our children's hospital. Children with coronavirus disease 2019 (COVID-19) infection or airborne illnesses, were not included in the audits. All other children, including those in other types of isolation, were included.

Project Design and Data Collection

QI Team

Team members included clinical nursing leaders, child life and music therapists, and a nursing QI leader. To begin, the group identified potential contributors to excessive screen time using a fishbone diagram (Supplemental Fig 6). Of the contributors, the group highlighted the lack of bedside alternatives and limited staff knowledge.

Outcome Measure and Audit Description

Baseline screen exposure was assessed by random audits performed by child life students. The audit was performed midday and documented utilization if screen media was on in the child's room. The audits started in November 2019. The baseline period, before significant interventions, occurred from November 2019 through August 2020.

When possible, the audits were completed at least once per week, though dependent on the student's schedule. The child life student went into all rooms that met inclusion criteria and used the opportunity to offer child life services if a caregiver was present. The audit recorded if a screen (TV or tablet) was on in the room and information on the room setting (Supplemental Fig 7). Some months in 2020 had lower census and audits were affected by COVID-19 isolation.

The primary outcome measure was percent of children who had screens turned on as measured by the audits. Although the audit did not assess how long the screen had been in use, this type of convenience and observational sample has been used successfully in other studies.[7,8]

Process Measures Obtained With Audit

The audits assessed process measures, including how often there was an adult present when the screen was on and if a screen alternative (ie, toy or mobile) was present in a child's room.

Process Measures Obtained With Staff Survey and Survey Description

Additional process measures included number of staff educated, the frequency that staff reported turning on screens for the target age group, and the frequency that staff reported offering screen alternatives to caregivers. To evaluate these measures, we surveyed direct care staff. The anonymous and voluntary survey was sent via e-mail and completed through a web-based survey tool. Survey responses were on a scale of 1 (never) to 5 (always). The survey respondents included nurses, nursing assistants, child life specialists, and music therapists. The survey assessed baseline behaviors and observations (Supplemental Fig 8).

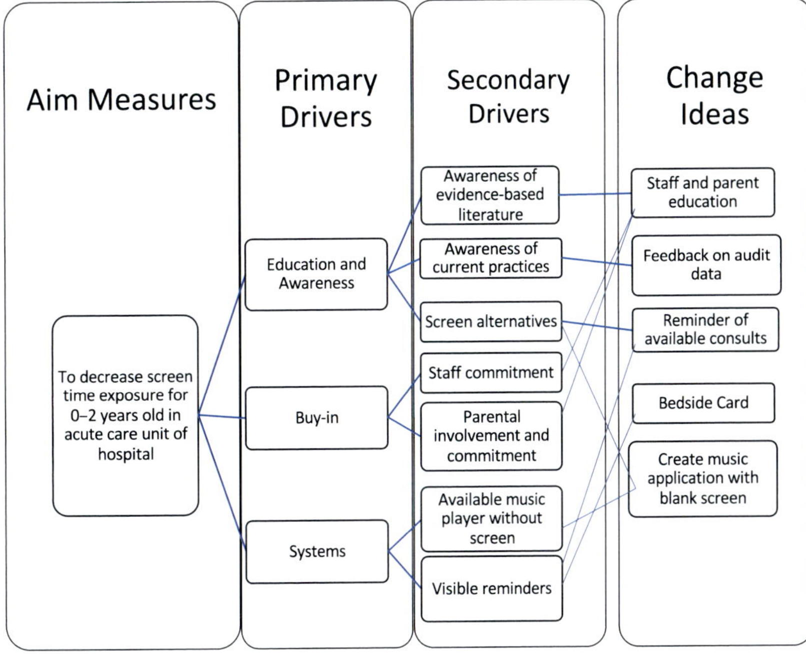

FIGURE 1 Key driver diagram outlining change ideas to limit digital screen exposure in hospitalized children.

Balancing Measures

The balancing measures evaluated potential reasons staff chose to use screens using survey questions about perceived workload when screens were used and if parents seemed upset when staff suggested turning off screens.

Interventions

The project interventions were established after review of the fishbone diagram and creation of a key driver diagram (Fig 1). The baseline survey results helped frame the following interventions: addition of a music application, bedside card for caregiver education, staff education, and staff reminder e-mail. The survey questions were written purposely to raise awareness of behaviors related to screens and help shape future interventions. The same survey was sent post intervention to assess for changes in behaviors and attitudes.

Before this project, when staff wanted to play music for children, they used the bedside tablet, which required concurrent viewing of an animated video. Once staff left the room, there was no control over subsequent content when the initially selected music finished. Our music therapy staff worked with an information technology consultant to develop an application for the existing tablet platform. This application played music with an accompanying blank screen. Evidence-based playlists were designed specifically for the infant and toddler age groups.[8,9] The music application automatically turned off after a set length of time, allowing staff to play age-appropriate music without screen exposure for a prescribed length of time.

The next intervention was designed to provide caregiver education about the AAP recommendations and available alternatives at our hospital with a small card at the bedside (Fig 2). This served as a reminder for staff to turn off screens and offer available alternatives.

Live education was provided to 35 nurses and nursing assistants. Those who could not attend received written materials. The education included baseline project data and promoted staff awareness of screen time alternatives including the new music application. The physicians, pediatric residents, and hospitalists were provided a similar presentation by the hospitalist lead. All staff were encouraged to educate caregivers on this initiative.

In summary, using a series of Plan Do Study Act cycles, our interventions started with the staff survey followed by the development of a music application as an alternative. We then supplied a bedside reminder for the staff in the form of a caregiver education card. Next, we used targeted staff education and reminded staff of the first 2 interventions, followed by a post intervention survey. After seeing an increase in screens being used in March 2021, we sent an e-mail to staff in April 2021 informing them of the audit data and reminding them to turn off screens.

Data Analysis and Statistical Analyses

The frequency of screen media turned on in the audited child's room was tracked by

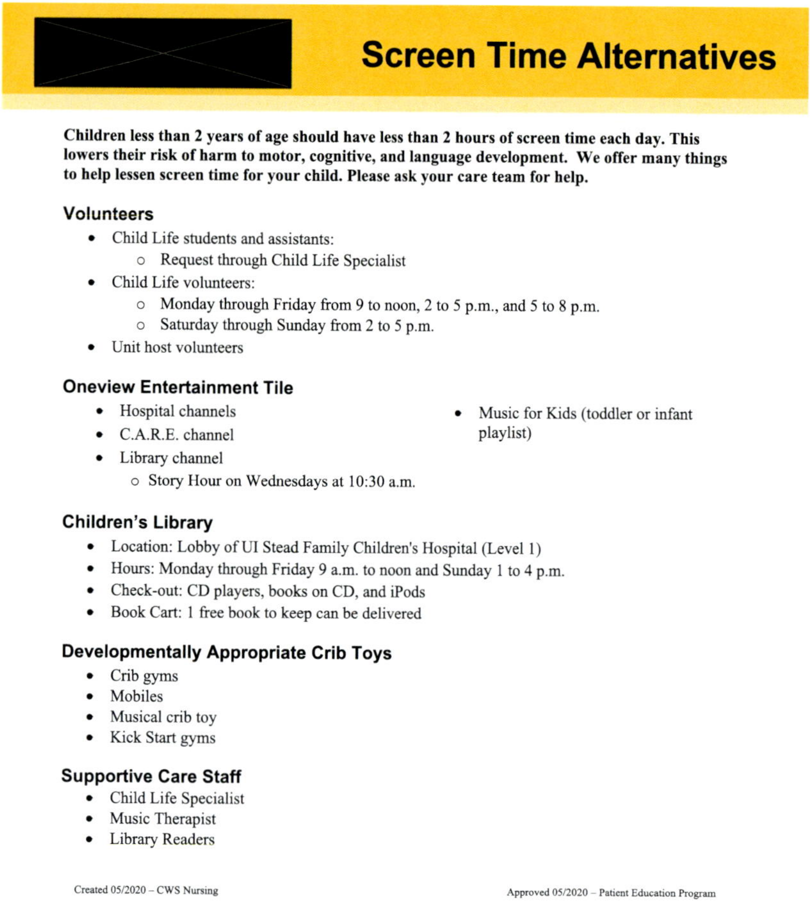

Screen Time Alternatives

Children less than 2 years of age should have less than 2 hours of screen time each day. This lowers their risk of harm to motor, cognitive, and language development. We offer many things to help lessen screen time for your child. Please ask your care team for help.

Volunteers

- Child Life students and assistants:
  - Request through Child Life Specialist
- Child Life volunteers:
  - Monday through Friday from 9 to noon, 2 to 5 p.m., and 5 to 8 p.m.
  - Saturday through Sunday from 2 to 5 p.m.
- Unit host volunteers

Oneview Entertainment Tile

- Hospital channels
- C.A.R.E. channel
- Library channel
  - Story Hour on Wednesdays at 10:30 a.m.
- Music for Kids (toddler or infant playlist)

Children's Library

- Location: Lobby of UI Stead Family Children's Hospital (Level 1)
- Hours: Monday through Friday 9 a.m. to noon and Sunday 1 to 4 p.m.
- Check-out: CD players, books on CD, and iPods
- Book Cart: 1 free book to keep can be delivered

Developmentally Appropriate Crib Toys

- Crib gyms
- Mobiles
- Musical crib toy
- Kick Start gyms

Supportive Care Staff

- Child Life Specialist
- Music Therapist
- Library Readers

Created 05/2020 – CWS Nursing   Approved 05/2020 – Patient Education Program

FIGURE 2 Bedside education card for caregivers listing digital screen alternatives.

month using a p-chart with control limits set at 3 standard deviations. Standard statistical quality control chart criteria were used for determining if observed changes were due to common cause variation or special-cause variation.[9] We generated the statistical process charts with QI-Charts from PIP Scoville Associates as an add-on for Microsoft Excel. The average values from the pre and post intervention process measures were compared with independent samples *t* test using Microsoft Excel, significance testing with $P < .05$.

RESULTS

A total of 700 audits were collected with an average of 41 audits per month. There were only 3 audits during November 2019 as the project was just starting, so these were combined with December 2019.

Primary Outcome

Month to month variation for screens turned on during audit is demonstrated with a statistical process control chart in Fig 3. The baseline period showed screens on for an average of 63% of audited children. Special cause was met after the intervention, demonstrated by a shift of 8 consecutive points below the center line.

Process Measures

Process Measures Obtained With Audits

The percent of audits with the screens on when an adult was present increased postintervention (67% vs 83% $P = .08$), special cause met with 2 out of 3 consecutive points at the upper confidence limit (Fig 4). Having a toy or mobile in place remained unchanged after interventions (43% vs 44%).

Process Measures Obtained With Staff Survey

Surveys were sent to staff members who provided direct patient care for the target population ($n = 60$). The survey respondents were mostly nurses (60%) and a combination of nursing assistants, occupational therapists, physical therapists, and child life specialists. The presurvey was completed by 25 staff members (42% response rate). The postsurvey was sent to the same staff group and 24 responded (40% response rate).

Comparison of the results of the pre and post survey are shown in Fig 5. In the pre survey, 84% of staff acknowledged that they turn on the TV at least sometimes, including 20% of staff that reported turning on the TV most of the time. In addition, 72% of staff reported parents always or most of the time turned on the TV. When parents have the TV on, 52% of staff reported that they never recommend turning it off. In the postintervention survey, most staff still reported turning on the TV at least sometimes, average responses in pre versus post of 2.4 vs 2.2 ($P = .31$). Notably, 0% reported this behavior most or all the time compared with 20% of staff preintervention. Fewer staff reported never recommending parents turn off the TV postintervention (52% vs 33%, $P = .16$). More staff reported offering parents screen alternatives postintervention (2.8 vs 3.4, $P = .10$).

Balancing Measures

Staff preintervention data revealed that 20% of staff felt that having the TV on made their job easier most or all the time compared with 13% after the intervention with average scores remaining largely unchanged (2.4 vs 2.3, $P = .72$). The perception of parents being upset stayed the same (2.3 vs 2.4, $P = .71$).

DISCUSSION

To our knowledge, this is the first QI initiative in the United States which aimed to reduce screen time exposure to young

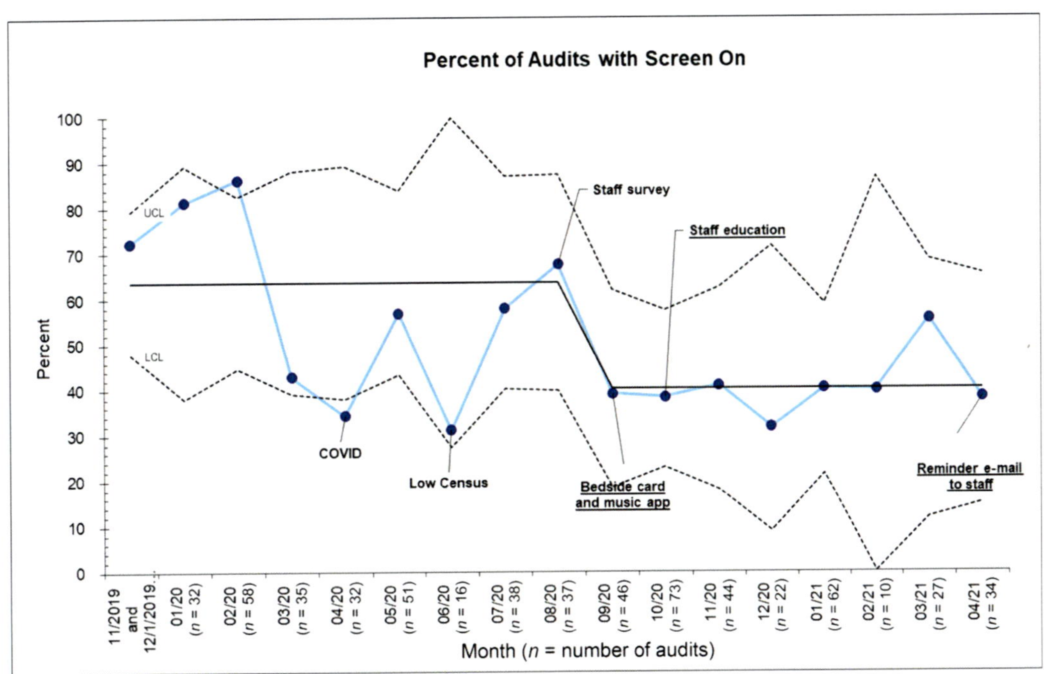

FIGURE 3 Percent of audits with screen on.

children in the hospital setting. The audits showed an overall reduction in screens used, though we did not achieve 50% reduction. It was encouraging to see the number of staff who reported turning on the TV "most of the time" was successfully reduced to zero. Despite the number of toy alternatives in the room remaining the same, staff reported offering more nonscreen alternatives to parents. Additionally, fewer staff reported that turning on the TV lessened their workload,

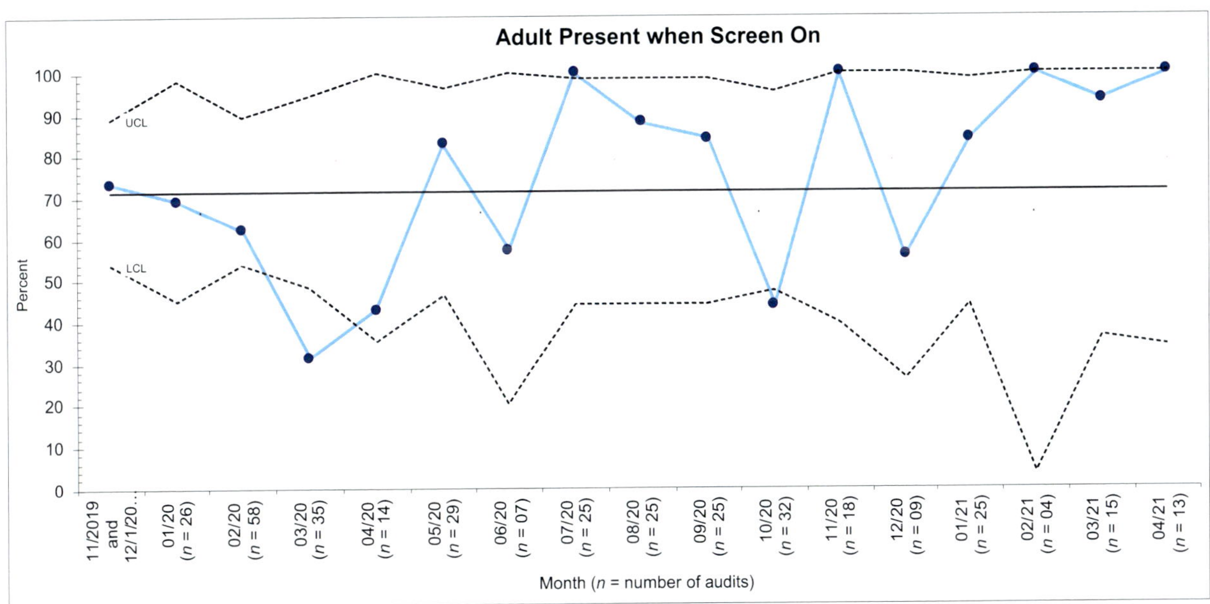

FIGURE 4 P-chart of process measure, percent of time an adult is present when screen is on during audit.

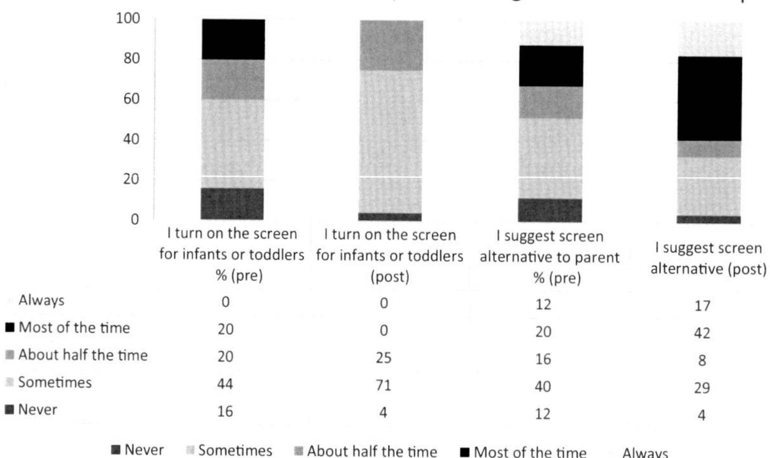

FIGURE 5 Survey results of health care staff perceptions of digital media use in the hospital.

though not statistically significant. The staff survey was intended to prompt staff to reflect on screen time behaviors as well as obtain data. Following the survey, we saw a decline in audits with screens on as our staff shifted their practice and modeled this to caregivers. The subsequent interventions helped keep this percentage lower than the baseline period. It does not appear that any 1 specific intervention resulted in improvement, rather a bundle of interventions implemented over time helped remind staff of the goal. TVs have long been a staple in hospital rooms, and now even more in-room tablets are making their way into children's hospitals around the country. It is unclear how many of these hospitals have provided staff and caregivers guidance on the optimal utilization of these devices for different age groups. The project prompted staff to reconsider screen utilization in young children by increasing their knowledge about the deleterious effects of screen time, as well as providing better screen alternatives. Playing certain recorded music for a set length of time has proven benefits in hospitalized pediatric patients.[10,11] Development of the music application was an important part of the project.

In the hospital, it is reasonable that caregivers may want to use screens while in the presence of their child. This project was not intended to eliminate this type of screen use. We wanted to educate caregivers and empower staff to turn off the screen when no adult was present to regulate the content and length of utilization. We saw an increase in the percent of time an adult was present when the screen was in use, which may indicate fewer screens were turned on or more turned off when no adult was present. This metric was important as these children cannot control the digital media. We thought it possible that perceived parental dissatisfaction may increase with more staff recommending turning off screens or decrease after the education interventions. However, this balancing measure remained unchanged.

Caregivers of children in the hospital are a captive audience to receive health maintenance counseling or generalized child safety messages. Hospitalizations may be an effective time to educate caregivers on topics not directly related to their child's diagnosis.[12] This is an opportunity to explain recommended guidelines for screen exposure and educate caregivers on the impact of excessive screen time on their child's development.[13] Additionally, as demonstrated repeatedly in safe sleep research, role modeling best practices for children while hospitalized is an essential element to influence caregiving practices in the home.14 Caregiving practices modeled by healthcare providers in the hospital are more likely to be adopted and continued in the home setting.[15]

This project's success was contingent on engaging front-line staff with effective education and providing alternatives to screen time. The project required engagement from child life specialists, music therapists, physicians, nurses, nursing assistants, and volunteers. Age-appropriate toys, puzzles, books, music, and interactions with caregivers or volunteers are all viable screen alternatives in the hospital. In our hospital, child life, music therapists, volunteers, and caregivers can be used to provide screen alternatives for young children. The COVID-19 pandemic limited volunteers in the hospital, however this project was conducted on a unit with very little volunteer support, so there was minimal impact on patients. Therapy services, toys, and books were still available. Not all hospitals have these resources and may need to find creative ways to engage caregivers in this initiative. In an Indian study, Singh et al were also able to demonstrate successful reduction in screen time for hospitalized children after implementation of a play protocol.[16]

We recognize that our project had limitations. This QI project took place in a single unit at a tertiary care hospital with specific digital media, which may limit generalizability. Not all hospitals have child life specialists, music therapists, and other staff dedicated to engaging children in their rooms. The audits were not consistent and were not representative of length of screen time exposure throughout the day, especially nights and weekends. Only the tablet and child's TV screen were assessed. The auditors did not collect data on phones or other screens. The audits did not capture children in airborne isolation, a population who may rely on screens more as they cannot leave the room. The bedside education card was only available in English. The staff survey sample size was relatively small and unmatched pre and post interventions. The survey results were subject to response bias and the postsurvey results may have been influenced by knowing the study aims.

CONCLUSIONS

Using QI methodology, we reduced screen time exposure in a vulnerable age group. We educated staff and caregivers about AAP recommendations and created an alternative music application. We hope modeling the use of screen alternatives will ultimately decrease screen exposure when the child goes home. The establishment of a consistent approach to screen media in the hospital setting could be a guide for other institutions to begin analyzing their own approach to technology utilization.

Implications

The impact of excessive screen time on children may lead to slower learning, decreased physical health and mobility, as well as shape a child's mental health. Using strategies to reduce screen exposure in the hospital, including modeling and education provided by hospital staff, could impact the public health of this generation of children for many years to come. Compliance has drifted slightly from 40% to 44% of screens on during random audits, which is still below the preproject baseline, despite the challenges of the ongoing pandemic. High levels of staff turnover, absence and use of traveling nurses coupled with increased staffing ratios have started to impact this process improvement effort.

Next Steps

To facilitate more compliance with the screen exposure guidelines, we will explore expansion of our volunteers and assure that all new and traveling staff are made aware of our standard. Future plans include implementation of this initiative on another acute care pediatric unit. Expanded implementation of a reliable standard throughout the children's hospital will facilitate consistent messaging from all hospital staff on the AAP recommendations.

Acknowledgments

We thank Micah Scott, IT consultant, for his help developing the music application; Lisa Miguel, Child Life Specialist, for her help with project interventions and audit gathering; and Kristen Nelson, Music Therapist, for her help in compiling the music playlists.

REFERENCES

1. Council on Communications and Media. Media and young minds. *Pediatrics.* 2016;138(5):e20162591
2. Hutton JS, Dudley J, Horowitz-Kraus T, DeWitt T, Holland SK. Associations between screen-based media use and brain white matter integrity in preschool-aged children. *JAMA Pediatr.* 2020;174(1):e193869
3. Anderson DR, Subrahmanyam K; Cognitive Impacts of Digital Media Workgroup. Cognitive impacts of digital media workgroup. digital screen media and cognitive development. *Pediatrics.* 2017;140(Suppl 2):S57–S61
4. Lissak G. Adverse physiological and psychological effects of screen time on children and adolescents: literature review and case study. *Environ Res.* 2018;164:149–157
5. Loprinzi PD, Davis RE. Secular trends in parent-reported television viewing among children in the United States, 2001-2012. *Child Care Health Dev.* 2016;42(2):288–291
6. Kabali HK, Irigoyen MM, Nunez-Davis R, et al. Exposure and use of mobile media devices by young children. *Pediatrics.* 2015;136(6):1044–1050
7. Arora G, Soares N, Li N, Zimmerman FJ. Screen media use in hospitalized children. *Hosp Pediatr.* 2016;6(5):297–304
8. DiMaggio DM, Sharif I, Hoffman-Rosenfeld J. TV guides: exposure of hospitalized children to inappropriate programming. *Ambul Pediatr.* 2003;3(2):98–101
9. Provost LP, Murray MS. *The health care data guide: Learning from data for improvement.* San Francisco, CA: Jossey-Bass; 2011
10. Hanson Abromeit D. The Newborn Individualized Developmental Care and Assessment Program (NIDCAP) as a model for clinical music therapy interventions with premature infants. *Music Ther Perspect.* 2003;21(2):60–68
11. Stouffer JW, Shirk BJ, Polomano RC. Practice guidelines for music interventions with hospitalized pediatric patients. *J Pediatr Nurs.* 2007;22(6):448–456
12. Winickoff JP, Hibberd PL, Case B, Sinha P, Rigotti NA. Child hospitalization: an opportunity for parental smoking intervention. *Am J Prev Med.* 2001;21(3): 218–220
13. Neophytou E, Manwell L, Eikelboom R. Effects of excessive screen time on neurodevelopment, learning, memory, mental health, and neurodegeneration: a scoping review. *Int J Ment Health Addict.* 2021;19:724–744
14. Goodstein MH, Bell T, Krugman SD. Improving infant sleep safety through a comprehensive hospital-based program. *Clin Pediatr (Phila).* 2015;54(3): 212–221

15. Newberry JA. Creating a safe sleep environment for the infant: what the pediatric nurse needs to know. *J Pediatr Nurs*. 2019;44:119–122

16. Singh V, Kalyan G, Saini SK, Bharti B, Malhi P. A quality improvement initiative to increase the opportunity of play activities and reduce the screen time among children admitted in hospital setting of a tertiary care centre, North India. *Indian J Pediatr*. 2021;88(1):9–15

Longitudinal Associations Between Screen Use and Reading in Preschool-Aged Children

Brae Anne McArthur, PhD,[a,b] Dillon Browne, PhD,[c] Sheila McDonald, PhD,[a,d] Suzanne Tough, PhD,[a,b,*] Sheri Madigan, PhD[a,b,*]

abstract

BACKGROUND AND OBJECTIVES: The home literacy environment has been identified as a key predictor of children's language, school readiness, academic achievement, and behavioral outcomes. With the increased accessibility and consumption of digital media, it is important to understand whether screen use impacts off-line enrichment activities such as reading or whether reading activities offset screen use. Using a prospective birth cohort, we examined reading and screen use at 24, 36, and 60 months to elucidate the directional association between screen use and reading over time.

METHODS: This study included data from 2440 mothers and children in Calgary, Alberta, drawn from the All Our Families cohort. Children's screen use and reading activities were assessed via maternal report at age 24, 36, and 60 months. Sociodemographic covariates were also collected.

RESULTS: Using a random-intercepts cross-lagged panel model, which statistically controls for individual-level confounds, this study revealed that greater screen use at 24 months was associated with lower reading at 36 months ($\beta = -.08$; 95% confidence interval: -0.13 to -0.02). In turn, lower reading at 36 months was associated with greater screen use at 60 months ($\beta = -.11$; 95% confidence interval: -0.19 to -0.02). Covariates did not modify the associations.

CONCLUSIONS: A reciprocal relationship between screen use and reading was identified. Early screen use was associated with lower reading activities, resulting in greater screen use at later ages. Findings emphasize the need for practitioners and educators to discuss screen use guidelines and encourage families to engage in device-free activities to foster early literacy exposure.

[a]University of Calgary, Calgary Alberta, Canada; [b]Alberta Children's Hospital Research Institute, Calgary, Alberta, Canada; [c]University of Waterloo, Waterloo, Ontario, Canada; and [d]Alberta Health Services, Calgary, Alberta, Canada

**Contributed equally as joint senior authors*

Drs McArthur and Madigan conceptualized and designed the study, conducted data analyses, drafted the manuscript, and reviewed and revised the manuscript; Dr Browne assisted with data analysis and reviewed the manuscript for important intellectual content; Drs McDonald and Tough conceptualized the cohort study, designed the data collection instruments and study methodology, secured funding for data collection, and reviewed the manuscript for important intellectual content; and all authors approved the final manuscript as submitted and agree to be accountable for all aspects of the work.

DOI: https://doi.org/10.1542/peds.2020-011429

Accepted for publication Feb 26, 2021

WHAT'S KNOWN ON THIS SUBJECT: Book reading is a critical element of the home environment that promotes school readiness and academic achievement. With increasing use of media devices, longitudinal research is needed to determine if screen use is interfering with off-line activities such as reading.

WHAT THIS STUDY ADDS: Findings support a dynamic relationship whereby screen use at 24 months leads to lower reading at 36 months, which in turn leads to greater screen use at 60 months. Families should be encouraged to engage in device-free time.

To cite: McArthur BA, Browne D, McDonald S, et al. Longitudinal Associations Between Screen Use and Reading in Preschool-Aged Children. *Pediatrics.* 2021; 147(6):e2020011429

ARTICLE

Children enter school with varying literacy skills, and these differences tend to get larger over time without intervention.[1,2] The home environment, including parent-child shared print book reading and language exposure, has been shown to have a large impact on children's later academic achievment.[3] In addition, shared book reading promotes important parent-child engagement during sensitive periods of development.[4] As a result, there have been long-standing efforts to identify factors that may influence the home literacy environment.[5–7]

With the increased use and accessibility of media devices,[8] screen use is becoming a consistent part of children's day-to-day lives. According to the displacement hypothesis,[9] when children are watching screens, they are less likely to spend time practicing skills important for learning and development.[10] As such, screen use may be influencing the home learning environment, specifically engagement in off-line enrichment activities such as reading print books,[11] and displacement may be one mechanism to explain the relation between screen time and delays in developmental skill acquisition. Although it is possible that screen use interrupts enriching off-line activities such as print book reading,[9,12] it is also possible that early reading activities may offset later screen use. However, to test this hypothesis, longitudinal data with repeated measurement are needed to examine directional associations between screen use and reading.

The primary aim of this study was to explicitly test what comes first: higher screen use or lower reading activities? In a sample of 2440 families, using a 3-wave (24, 36, and 60 months) random intercept cross-lagged panel model (RI-CLPM),[13] we predict that higher screen use will relate to lower reading activities at later time points. The RI-CLPM is considered to be the most robust method for addressing directionality in observational studies by statistically controlling for individual-level confounds, such as stable family-level stressors.[13] The secondary aim of this study was to explore the extent to which the longitudinal associations between screen use and reading varied on the basis of sociodemographic covariates. Implications of these findings could inform pediatricians, health care practitioners, child care providers, educators and policymakers seeking to guide parents on appropriate recommendations for screen exposure and off-line activities such as reading during the sensitive period of early childhood.

METHODS

Study Design and Population

Participants were from All Our Families, a pregnancy cohort of 3388 mothers and children from Calgary, Canada.[14,15] Women were recruited between August 2008 and December 2010 through primary health care offices, community advertising, and laboratories. Inclusion criteria were (1) age ≥18 years, (2) fluent in English, (3) gestational age <25 weeks, and (4) receiving community-based prenatal care. Mothers were followed-up at <25 weeks' gestation and at 4, 12, 24, 36, and 60 months' postpartum. The 24-, 36-, and 60-month time points were the focus of this analysis because screen use and reading variables were both collected. A detailed description of the study sample can be found in Table 1. All procedures were approved by the institutional ethics board.

Measures

Screen Use

When children were aged 24, 36, and 60 months, mothers reported the range of time their child spent using electronic devices (ie, watching television programs; watching movies, videos, or stories on a videocassette recorder or digital video disk player; and using a computer, gaming system, or other screen-based device) on a typical weekday and typical weekend day. A weighted average across week and weekend days and electronic devices was calculated to yield screen use in hours per week. At each time point, outliers >4 SDs from the mean were winsorized[16] (n = 8 at 24 months, n = 16 at 36 months, and n = 7 at 60 months).

Reading Activities

When children were aged 24, 36, and 60 months, mothers reported the range of time their child spent in reading activities using a 4-point response scale. At 24 months, mothers were asked, "Do you or another adult of the household read to your child or show him/her picture books?" with response options ranging from (1) never to (4) daily. At 36 months, mothers were asked, "How many minutes each day do you spend sharing books with your child? " with response options ranging from (1) 0 to 10 minutes to (4) ≥30 minutes. At 60 months, mothers were asked, "How many hours per day does your child spend doing the following activities outside of child care, preschool, or school: Read or look at books?" on a typical weekday and weekend day. Response options ranged from (1) none or 0 minutes to (4) ≥3 hours. At 60 months, a weighted average across week and weekend days was calculated to yield reading in hours per day, with a range from (1) none or 0 minutes to (4) ≥3 hours. The reading items were designed to reflect the natural progression of reading activities across early childhood. Results from this study suggest consistency in this measurement method over time (24–36 months [β = .23; 95% confidence interval (CI): .18 to .29]; 36–60 months [β = .24; 95% CI: .18 to .29]).

TABLE 1 Sample Demographics and Study Characteristics

Characteristic	Value
Maternal education, *n* (%)	
Less than high school	40 (1.6)
Graduated high school	104 (4.3)
Some college or trade school or university	233 (9.6)
Graduated college or trade school or university	1265 (51.9)
Some graduate school	42 (1.7)
Completed graduate school	307 (12.6)
Missing	449 (18.3)
Household income, CAD $, *n* (%)	
≤29 999	35 (1.4)
30 000–39 999	43 (1.8)
40 000–49 999	50 (2.1)
50 000–59 999	98 (4.0)
60 000–69 999	76 (3.1)
70 000–79 999	122 (5.0)
80 000–89 999	140 (5.7)
90 000–99 999	147 (6.0)
100 000–124 999	358 (14.7)
125 000–149 999	258 (10.6)
≥150 000	644 (26.4)
Missing	469 (19.1)
Maternal race and/or ethnicity, *n* (%)	
White	1993 (81.7)
Black and/or African American	29 (1.2)
Indigenous	12 (0.5)
Asian	254 (10.4)
Latin American	37 (1.5)
Multiracial or other	100 (4.1)
Missing	15 (0.6)
Child sex, *n* (%)	
Female	937 (38.4)
Male	1018 (41.7)
Missing	485 (19.9)
Nonparental child care or day care before 60 mo, *n* (%)	
Yes	1433 (58.8)
No	533 (21.9)
Missing	474 (19.4)
Maternal screen use at 24 mo, *n* (%)	
None	111 (4.6)
<1 h	441 (18.1)
1–<3 h	859 (35.3)
3–<5 h	149 (6.1)
5–<7 h	24 (1.0)
≥7 h	10 (0.4)
Missing	846 (34.6)
Maternal reading at 24 mo, *n* (%)	
None	199 (8.2)
<1 h	879 (36.1)
1–<3 h	440 (18.1)
3–<5 h	57 (2.3)
5–<7 h	13 (0.5)
≥7 h	6 (0.2)
Missing	846 (34.6)
Attended the library at 24 mo, *n* (%)	
Yes	961 (39.5)
No	635 (26.0)
Missing	844 (34.5)
Problem behavior (BITSEA) at 24 mo, *n* (%)	
At risk	236 (9.7)
Normative	1344 (55.1)
Missing	860 (35.2)

Covariates

Child sex (1 [female]; 0 [male]), household income (reported in increments of $10 000 Canadian dollars [CAD]: 1 [≤$29 999]; 11 [≥$150 000]), and maternal education (1 [less than a high school education]; 6 [completed graduate school]) were maternal self-report. At 24 months, maternal screen use and maternal reading were measured with single self-report items asking the amount of time mothers spend watching television or reading, respectively, on a typical weekday (1 [none]; 6 [≥7 hours per day]). Attending the library (eg, story time, borrowing books or videos, etc) in the past year (yes [1]; no [0]) was also measured with a single self-report item. Mothers completed the Brief Infant-Toddler Social and Emotional Assessment (BITSEA) to identify child behavior problems (eg, aggression, defiance, over-activity, negative emotionality, anxiety, and withdrawal). By using the BITSEA standardized scoring cutoffs, children were categorized with possible behavioral problems if they scored in the ≥75th percentile on the scale.[17] At 60 months, mothers responded to "has your child been in nonparental child care or day care on a regular basis before this year?" (0 [no]; 1 [yes]).

Statistical Analyses

The longitudinal associations between hours of screen use and reading activities were examined by using an RI-CLPM.[13] The RI-CLPM statistically distinguishes variance at the temporal level (ie, within-person or time-varying) from variance at the individual level (ie, between-person or stable) and, therefore, constitutes a multilevel approach accounting for repeated measurements that are nested within individuals. An important advantage of the RI-CLPM over the common cross-lagged panel model is that RI-CLPM controls for

TABLE 1 Continued

Characteristic	Value
Weekly hours of screen use at 24 mo, mean (SD)	17.07 (11.82)
Weekly hours of screen use at 36 mo, mean (SD)	24.90 (12.50)
Weekly hours of screen use at 60 mo, mean (SD)	10.84 (5.29)
Reading activities at 24 mo, mean (SD)	3.92 (0.29)
Reading activities at 36 mo, mean (SD)	2.61 (0.94)
Reading activities at 60 mo, mean (SD)	2.48 (0.52)

stable individuals' differences (ie, between-person and time-invariant effects, such as stable family-level stressors) in reading activities and screen use, allowing for greater insight into how the two central constructs in the model (ie, screen use and reading activities) are linked at an intraindividual (ie, within-person and time-varying) level. This approach has been shown to reduce bias in directional estimates and more closely approximate causal relationships.[18]

First, the standard RI-CLPM was estimated. In the RI-CLPM, between-person (stable) factors were extracted from the repeated measures of screen use and reading, and these factors were permitted to covary. The within-person component comprises 3 types of estimates: (1) autoregressions (ie, lags) capture the within-person, rank-order stability in constructs over time; (2) within-time covariances capture the strength and direction of associations between screen use and reading within persons at each time point; and (3) the cross lags capture the longitudinal and directional associations between screen use and reading within persons and are comparable to the proportion of unique variance explained in the outcome that is not shared with any other predictor (ie, a squared semipartial correlation[19,20]; Fig 1). After fitting the standard RI-CLPM, pairwise comparisons were conducted by using post hoc t tests to identify the extent to which the cross-lag estimates varied between different levels of the covariates (measured at the between-person level). Statistical significance was set at the $P < .05$, 2-tailed level; 95% CIs are reported. All analyses were conducted in Mplus version 8.1.[21]

Missing Data

From the initial pregnancy cohort ($N = 3388$), 95% ($n = 3223$) agreed to be contacted for follow-up research. Of those who agreed to follow-up and were eligible at the time of questionnaire completion, 76% completed the 24-month questionnaire ($n = 1595$), 69% completed the 36-month questionnaire ($n = 1994$), and 71% completed the 60-month questionnaire ($n = 1992$). Attrition rates observed in the current study are similar to other prospective birth cohorts.[22–24] Predictors of dropout are reported elsewhere (younger mothers and lower income).[10] Consistent with other pediatric RI-CLPMs,[10] participants were included ($n = 2440$) if they completed questionnaires for at least 1 time point at either 24, 36, or 60 months. To adjust for missing data, models were run with full-information maximum likelihood estimation.[25,26]

RESULTS

Primary Analyses

The standard RI-CLPM (Fig 1) revealed that the model was a good fit to the observed data on the basis of fit indices ($\chi^2_1 = 0.09$; $P = .768$; root mean square error of approximation = 0.00; 95% CI: 0.00 to 0.04; comparative fit index = 1.00; standardized root mean square residual = 0.002).

In the time-variant component of the model, statistically significant autocorrelations for every estimated lag indicate substantial within-person stability in constructs over time. That is, on average, children's screen use and reading activities were stable across adjacent time points. As detailed in Fig 1 and Table 2, after accounting for this temporal stability, there was a significant and negative cross lag linking higher levels of screen use at 24 months of age with lower levels of reading activities at 36 months of age ($\beta = -.08$; 95% CI: $-.13$ to $-.02$). The obverse direction of higher levels of reading activities at 24 months being associated with lower exposure to screens at 36 months was not observed ($\beta = -.05$; 95% CI: $-.11$ to .01). At 36 months of age, lower levels of reading activities predicted higher exposure to screen use at 60 months ($\beta = -.11$; 95% CI: $-.19$ to $-.02$). The obverse association was not observed ($\beta = .01$; 95% CI: $-.04$ to .06). Also, within-time covariances were significant at 24 and 36 months but not at 60 months, suggesting that, on average, at the 24- and 36-month study waves, children's screen use was significantly related to children's reading activities ($\beta = -.10$ [95% CI: $-.17$ to $-.04$] and $\beta = -.08$ [95% CI: $-.13$ to $-.03$], respectively).

Taken together, these findings suggest that higher levels of screen use at 24 months of age, relative to a child's average level of screen use (ie, the child's stable mean), was associated with significantly lower levels of reading activities at the next study wave, relative to a child's average level of reading. In addition, lower levels of reading activities at 36 months of age, relative to a child's average level of reading, was associated with significantly higher levels of screen use at 60 months of age, relative to a child's average level of screen use.

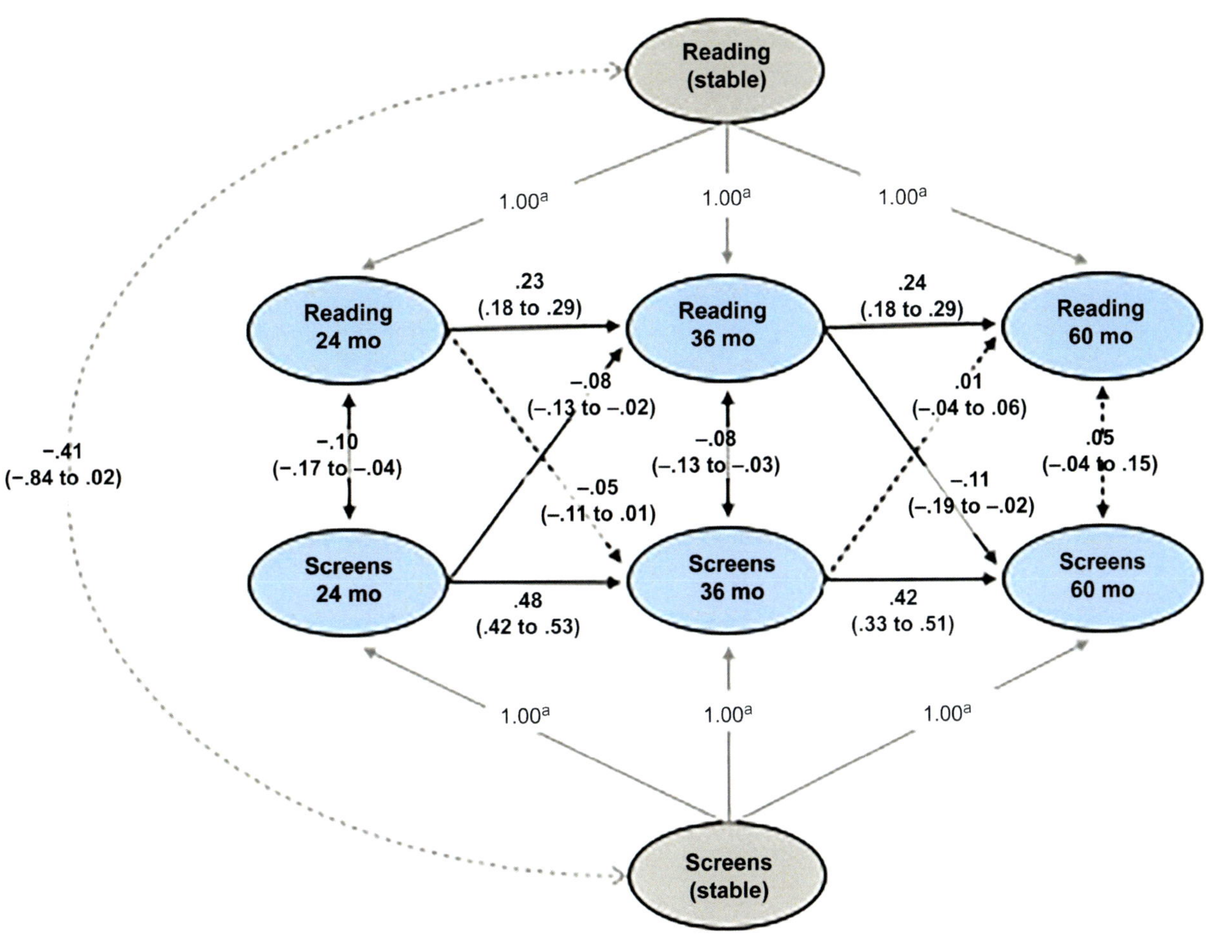

FIGURE 1

The standard RI-CLPM revealing within-person association between screen use and reading from ages 24 to 60 months, controlling for between-person differences. Standardized estimates (β) and 95% CIs are presented. Solid lines represent estimates in which 95% CIs do not include 0. The central, blue-tinted part of the model is the within-person (dynamic) part, and the outer, gray-tinted part of the model is the between-person (stable) component.
[a] Pathways constrained to 1.00 to extract between-person factor (n = 2440).

Secondary Analyses

To determine the extent to which the longitudinal associations between screen use and reading varied on the basis of covariates, the differences in the cross-lagged associations between levels of each study covariate were examined (Table 3). Cross-lagged parameters did not significantly differ on the basis of different levels of the study covariates.

DISCUSSION

With expanding media options and a dynamic digital landscape, screen use is a common household activity for young children.[8] With this change comes growing concern about the role of screen use on the home learning environment, specifically engagement in off-line enrichment activities such as print book reading. This longitudinal, 3-wave study uses repeated measures and a rigorous statistical model that more closely approximate causality to clarify whether screen use interferes with later print book reading or if early reading activities may offset later screen use. Results suggest that higher screen use at 24 months is related to lower reading activities at 36 months, and in turn, lower reading activities at 36 months is associated with greater screen use at 60 months. The obverse associations (ie, greater reading at 24 months leading to lower screen time at 36 months and, in turn, greater reading at 60 months) were not observed.

A robust body of literature underscores the importance of the early home learning environment to encourage the development of school readiness and literacy skills.[5,23] Consistent with the displacement hypothesis,[9] this study provides support for the notion that screen use may be interfering with reading activities. Indeed, at 24 months, it

TABLE 2 Standardized and Unstandardized Autoregressive and Cross-Lagged Coefficients From the Standard RI-CLPM

Paths	β (95% CI)[a]	B (95% CI)[b]
Autoregressive parameters		
Screen time, mo		
24 → 36	.48 (.42 to .53)[c]	.51 (.43 to .59)[c]
36 → 60	.42 (.33 to .51)[c]	.12 (.07 to .17)[c]
Reading, mo		
24 → 36	.23 (.18 to .29)[c]	.79 (.61 to .97)[c]
36 → 60	.24 (.18 to .29)[c]	.13 (.09 to .16)[c]
Cross-lagged parameters		
Screen time → reading, mo		
24 → 36	−.08 (−.13 to −.02)[c]	−.01 (−.01 to −.002)[c]
36 → 60	.01 (−.04 to .06)	.00 (−.002 to .003)
Reading → screen time, mo		
24 → 36	−.05 (−.11 to .01)	−2.24 (−4.80 to .32)
36 → 60	−.11 (−.19 to −.02)[c]	−.39 (−.67 to −.11)[c]

B, unstandardized β coefficient; β, standardized β coefficient; →, predicting.

[a] Standardized β coefficients represent the SD change in an outcome variable (eg, reading at 36 mo) associated with a 1 SD change in the predictor (eg, screen time at 24 mo).

[b] Unstandardized B coefficients represent the unit change in an outcome variable (eg, 1 level of reading at 36 mo) associated with a unit change in the predictor (eg,1 hour of screen time at 24 mo).

[c] Estimates in which 95% CIs do not include 0.

was observed that greater screen use per week relates to a lower level of reading activities at 36 months. In addition, through interpretation of the unstandardized coefficients, a 10-minute decrease in reading per day at 36 months of age relates to a ~25-minute increase in screen use per week at 60 months of age. These findings highlight a reciprocal process between screen use and reading that unfolds over time, in which screen use negatively influences reading activities and then lowered reading activities lead to greater screen use.

With the increased use and accessibility of media devices, families may turn to electronics to promote reading. Although reading electronic books was not examined herein, researchers have recently found that, for preschool-aged children, parents and children tend to collaborate and verbalize less when reading electronic books in comparison with reading print books.[27,28] Overall, there appears to be less reciprocity and conversational turns (specific elements of the early reading environment known to promote language learning and literacy skills) when using electronic books,[4] and thus encouraging reading activities that involve print books for young children may be advised.

Although past research supports that many factors in the home environment influence screen use[29] and reading activities,[4,5] results from the post hoc analysis of covariates reveal that the sociodemographic variables included in this study did not significantly modify the magnitude of the associations between screen use and reading over time. This finding suggests that sociodemographic factors may be more influential at a between-person level (eg, when predicting overall screen use or reading activities for different children) but may be less impactful at a within-person level (eg, impacting the associations between reading and screen use over time for a specific child).

A number of practice and policy implications arise from this study. Most importantly, this study highlights the need for practitioners, health care workers, parents, policymakers, and educators to promote adherence to screen use guidelines. This is especially important because up to 95% of preschoolers are exceeding the current screen use guidelines[30] of no more than 1 hour of screen time daily.[31] Family media plans[32] can be devised to help families develop healthy media habits. Early discussions with family may be critical because research reveals that once problematic screen use habits are developed, they tend to persist over the early childhood period.[33] On the basis of the within-person stability of shared reading and screen media habits starting at 24 months of age, this study also emphasizes the importance of establishing early reading routines known to be foundational for child development and learning and reaffirms the need for early discussion of reading in pediatric offices. These discussions can focus on the 5 R's[34] of early learning: reading together every day; rhyme and play; developing consistent sleep, eating, reading and play routines; reward with praise; and nurture relationships rich in serve and return interactions. At a policy level, increased access to books, programs designed to help connect at risk-families with literary resources (eg, reach out and read[35]), broader dissemination of screen use guidelines for children aged <5 years, and a combination of early interventions targeted at both reading and screen use habits are needed.

Using a large cohort and a longitudinal research design, as well as a robust statistical method, this study sheds light on the direction of the association between screen use and reading activities across early childhood. However, the findings must be interpreted with the following limitations in mind. First, this study included a predominantly high-income, highly educated sample of participants, which may limit generalizability to other populations. Second, the method of measurement used for screen use did not capture the content (eg, educational programing) or context (eg, solitary versus coviewing) of screen use.

TABLE 3 Differences in the Cross-Lagged Associations Linking Screen Use and Reading, by Covariates

Paths	Difference (95% CI)[a]	
	Income[b]	Education[c]
Screen time → reading, mo		
24 → 36	0.00 (−0.01 to 0.01)	0.01 (−0.004 to 0.02)
36 → 60	0.00 (−0.01 to 0.01)	0.00 (−0.004 to 0.01)
Reading → screen time, mo		
24 → 36	−0.55 (−7.39 to 6.28)	2.33 (−3.32 to 7.97)
36 → 60	−0.66 (−1.64 to 0.32)	−0.11 (−0.83 to 0.62)
	Maternal reading[d]	Maternal screen use[e]
Screen time → reading, mo		
24 → 36	0.00 (−0.01 to 0.01)	0.00 (−0.01 to 0.01)
36 → 60	−0.01 (−0.01 to 0.00)	0.01 (−0.001 to 0.01)
Reading → screen time, mo		
24 → 36	−3.93 (−9.50 to 1.65)	4.44 (−1.39 to 10.27)
36 → 60	0.14 (−0.55 to 0.83)	−0.20 (−1.46 to 1.05)
	Problem behavior[f]	Child sex[g]
Screen time → reading, mo		
24 → 36	0.01 (−0.01 to 0.02)	−0.01 (−0.02 to 0.004)
36 → 60	0.00 (−0.01 to 0.01)	0.00 (−0.001 to 0.005)
Reading → screen time, mo		
24 → 36	1.41 (−5.28 to 8.10)	0.89 (−4.78 to 6.53)
36 → 60	−0.31 (−1.21 to 0.59)	−0.33 (−0.88 to 0.22)
	Child care[h]	Access to library[i]
Screen time → reading, mo		
24 → 36	0.00 (−0.01 to 0.01)	0.01 (−0.003 to 0.02)
36 → 60	0.01 (−0.001 to 0.01)	0.01 (−0.001 to 0.01)
Reading → screen time, mo		
24 → 36	1.13 (−4.58 to 6.84)	0.17 (−5.00 to 5.33)
36 → 60	−0.26 (−0.94 to 0.42)	−0.17 (−0.87 to 0.52)

→, predicting.

a Difference in the cross-lagged associations by covariate group.

b Defined as low income (CAD$ <60 000; 1) and high income (CAD$ ≥60 000; 0).

c Defined as lower education (some high school, graduated high school, and some postsecondary; 1) and higher education (graduated postsecondary, some graduate school, and completed graduate school; 0).

d Defined as low maternal reading (below median; 1) and high maternal reading (at or above median; 0).

e Defined as low maternal screen use (below median; 1) and high maternal screen use (at or above median; 0).

f Defined as at risk (at or above the cutoff score on the BITSEA problem behavior scale; 1) and normative (below the cutoff score on the BITSEA problem behavior scale; 0).

g Defined as male (1) and female (0).

h Defined as nonparental child care or day care (1) and other (0).

i Defined as attending the library (1) and not attending the library (0).

Presumably, families vary on the content and context in which screens are used, and these elements of screen use may have a different association with language and literacy.[36] Third, although this study reveals an association between screen use and reading, further research is needed to determine the specific threshold at which screen use influences reading. Fourth, because of the rapid progression of technology, exposure and accessibility to screens may have changed over the course of this multiwave study.[8] Additionally, although parents are arguably the best informants of child activities between 24 and 60 months, single-informant measurement introduces the potential for bias. With regards to reading, a single item was used to capture the frequency of reading activities at each time point. Although the reading items were designed to reflect the natural progression of reading activities across early childhood, single-item measurement at each time point provides fewer points of discrimination and potentially limits the sensitivity, or variation, in the measure. This study would be strengthened by more detailed measurement of the home reading environment, including parent literacy skills and objective measures of parent-child shared reading experiences (eg, conversational turns, parent engagement, etc).

CONCLUSIONS

With the increased exposure to digital media, screen use is now a regular part of children's day-to-day lives. In response to this increase in exposure, there is a critical need to understand how screen use may be influencing the home learning environment, specifically engagement in off-line enrichment activities such as reading. This study provides support for a reciprocal relationship between screen use and reading activities. Higher screen use at 24 months of age related to lower reading activities at 36 months of age, and in turn, lower levels of reading at 36 months of age related to higher levels of screen use at the next time point. The findings from this study support the need for practitioners, child care professionals, and educators to encourage families to engage in healthy use of screen devices (ie, limited duration) and to encourage device-free time to establish early reading habits.

ACKNOWLEDGMENTS

We acknowledge the contributions of the All Our Families research team and thank the participants who took part in the study.

ABBREVIATIONS

BITSEA: Brief Infant-Toddler Social and Emotional Assessment
CAD: Canadian dollar
CI: confidence interval
RI-CLPM: random intercept cross-lagged panel model

Address correspondence to Sheri Madigan, PhD, Department of Psychology, University of Calgary, 2500 University Ave, Calgary, AB, Canada T2N 1N4. E-mail: sheri.madigan@ucalgary.ca

PEDIATRICS (ISSN Numbers: Print, 0031-4005; Online, 1098-4275).

FINANCIAL DISCLOSURE: The authors have indicated they have no financial relationships relevant to this article to disclose.

FUNDING: Supported by Alberta Innovates Health Solutions Interdisciplinary Team grant 200700595, the Alberta Children's Hospital Foundation, and the Max Bell Foundation. The principal investigator of the All Our Families Study is Dr Tough. Research support was provided to Dr Madigan and Dr. Browne by the Canada Research Chairs program. Dr McArthur was supported by a fellowship from the Alberta Children's Hospital Research Institute.

POTENTIAL CONFLICT OF INTEREST: The authors have indicated they have no potential conflicts of interest to disclose.

COMPANION PAPER: A companion to this article can be found online at www.pediatrics.org/cgi/doi/10.1542/peds.2020-047472.

REFERENCES

1. Stanovich KE. Matthew effects in reading: some consequences of individual differences in the acquisition of literacy. *Read Res Q*. 1986;21(4): 360–407
2. NICHD Early Child Care Research Network. Early child care and children's development prior to school entry: results from the NICHD study of early child care. *Am Educ Res J*. 2002;39(1): 133–164
3. Barnes E, Puccioni J. Shared book reading and preschool children's academic achievement: evidence from the Early Childhood Longitudinal Study-Birth cohort. *Infant Child Dev*. 2017; 26(6):e2035
4. Duursma E, Augustyn M, Zuckerman B. Reading aloud to children: the evidence. *Arch Dis Child*. 2008;93(7):554–557
5. Tamis-LeMonda CS, Luo R, McFadden KE, Bandel ET, Vallotton C. Early home learning environment predicts children's 5th grade academic skills. *Appl Dev Sci*. 2019;23(2):153–169
6. Johnson AD, Martin A, Brooks-Gunn J, Petrill SA. Order in the house! Associations among household chaos, the home literacy environment, maternal reading ability, and children's early reading. *Merrill Palmer Q (Wayne State Univ Press)*. 2008;54(4):445–472
7. Greenwood P, Hutton J, Dudley J, Horowitz-Kraus T. Maternal reading fluency is associated with functional connectivity between the child's future reading network and regions related to executive functions and language processing in preschool-age children. *Brain Cogn*. 2019;131:87–93
8. Rideout V. *The Common Sense Census: Media Use by Kids Zero to Eight*. San Francisco, CA: Common Sense Media; 2017
9. Christakis DA. The effects of infant media usage: what do we know and what should we learn? *Acta Paediatr*. 2009;98(1):8–16
10. Madigan S, Browne D, Racine N, Mori C, Tough S. Association between screen time and children's performance on a developmental screening test. *JAMA Pediatr*. 2019;173(3):244–250
11. McArthur BA, Eirich R, McDonald S, Tough S, Madigan S. Screen use relates to decreased offline enrichment activities. *Acta Paediatr*. 2021;110(3): 896–898
12. Radesky JS, Schumacher J, Zuckerman B. Mobile and interactive media use by young children: the good, the bad, and the unknown. *Pediatrics*. 2015;135(1): 1–3
13. Hamaker EL, Kuiper RM, Grasman RPPP. A critique of the cross-lagged panel model. *Psychol Methods*. 2015;20(1): 102–116
14. Tough SC, McDonald SW, Collisson BA, et al. Cohort profile: the all our babies pregnancy cohort (AOB). *Int J Epidemiol*. 2017;46(5):1389–1390k
15. McDonald SW, Lyon AW, Benzies KM, et al. The All Our Babies Pregnancy Cohort: Design, Methods, and Participant Characteristics. In: *BMC Pregnancy Childbirth*, vol. 13. 2013:S2
16. Berry KJ, Johnston JE, Mielke PWJ. *A Chronicle of Permutation Statistical Methods: 1920–2000, and Beyond*. New York, NY: Springer; 2014
17. Briggs-Gowan MJ, Carter AS, Irwin JR, Wachtel K, Cicchetti DV. The Brief Infant-Toddler Social and Emotional Assessment: screening for social-emotional problems and delays in competence. *J Pediatr Psychol*. 2004; 29(2):143–155
18. Berry D, Willoughby MT. On the practical interpretability of cross-lagged panel models: rethinking a developmental workhorse. *Child Dev*. 2017;88(4): 1186–1206
19. Schuurman NK, Ferrer E, de Boer-Sonnenschein M, Hamaker EL. How to compare cross-lagged associations in a multilevel autoregressive model. *Psychol Methods*. 2016;21(2):206–221
20. Tabachnick BG, Fidell LS. *Using Multivariate Statistics*. Harlow, United Kingdom: Pearson Education; 2014
21. Muthén L, Muthén B. *Mplus Statistical Modeling Software: Release 8.0*. Los Angeles, CA: Muthén & Muthén; 2017
22. National Institute of Child Health and Human Development Early Child Care Research Network. Duration and developmental timing of poverty and children's cognitive and social development from birth through third grade. *Child Dev*. 2005;76(4):795–810
23. Browne DT, Wade M, Prime H, Jenkins JM. School readiness amongst urban Canadian families: risk profiles and family mediation. *J Educ Psychol*. 2018; 110(1):133–146
24. Sontag-Padilla L, Burns RM, Shih RA, et al. *The Urban Child Institue CANDLE*

Study. Santa Monica, CA: Rand Corporation; 2015

25. Graham JW. Missing data analysis: making it work in the real world. *Annu Rev Psychol.* 2009;60:549–576
26. Yuan KH, Bentler PM. 5. Three likelihood-based methods for mean and covariance structure analysis with nonnormal missing data. *Sociol Methodol.* 2000;30(1):165–200
27. Munzer TG, Miller AL, Weeks HM, Kaciroti N, Radesky J. Differences in parent-toddler interactions with electronic versus print books. *Pediatrics.* 2019;143(4):e20182012
28. Munzer TG, Miller AL, Weeks HM, Kaciroti N, Radesky J. Parent-toddler social reciprocity during reading from electronic tablets vs print books. *JAMA Pediatr.* 2019;173(11):1–8
29. Browne D, Thompson DA, Madigan S. Digital media use in children: clinical vs scientific responsibilities. *JAMA Pediatr.* 2020;174(2):111–112
30. Madigan S, Racine N, Tough S. Prevalence of preschoolers meeting vs exceeding screen time guidelines. *JAMA Pediatr.* 2019;174(1):93–95
31. American Academy of Pediatrics. American Academy of Pediatrics announces new recommendations for children's media use. 2016. Available at: https://services.aap.org/en/news-room/news-releases/aap/2016/aap-announces-new-recommendations-for-media-use. Accessed September 12, 2018
32. American Academy of Pediatrics. Family media plan. 2019. Available at: https://www.healthychildren.org/English/media/Pages/default.aspx?gclid=EAIaIQobChMIoq2F-eiA3QIVUFuGCh3e0gDnEAAYBCAAEgJqNPD_BwE. Accessed July 8, 2019
33. McArthur BA, Browne D, Tough S, Madigan S. Trajectories of screen use during early childhood: predictors and associated behavior and learning outcomes. *Comput Human Behav.* 2020; 113:106501
34. American Academy of Pediatrics. Early education - The 5 R's. Available at: https://www.aap.org/en-us/advocacy-and-policy/aap-health-initiatives/EBCD/Pages/Five.aspx. Accessed October 23, 2020
35. Klass P, Dreyer BP, Mendelsohn AL. Reach out and read: literacy promotion in pediatric primary care. *Adv Pediatr.* 2009;56(1):11–27
36. Madigan S, McArthur BA, Anhorn C, Eirich R, Christakis DA. Associations between screen use and child language skills: a systematic review and meta-analysis. *JAMA Pediatr.* 2020;174(7): 665–675

Establishing Early Literacy Habits in a Profit-Driven Digital World

Jenny S. Radesky, MD

Books are remarkable objects. They carry children into imaginary spaces and offer parents a familiar script to settle children down at night. Books challenge readers' minds to stretch their attention span, pause and contemplate, and take others' perspectives. Early book sharing is promoted by the American Academy of Pediatrics because of its clear impact on reading scores, which predict high school graduation rates.[1]

Since the introduction of television, early childhood experts have wondered whether time spent in pleasurable but "minds-off" screen experiences displaces reading. Studies using time use diaries and surveys offered conflicting evidence[2,3] but suggested that educational television was linked with more reading in stressed families.[4]

However, the digital ecosystem has changed dramatically in the past two decades. Children can find their favorite programs on demand in any room of the house or moment of boredom. Myriad digital products marketed to children provide engaging interactivity but often have low educational value and high advertising load.[5] By algorithmically predicting what children might click on next, platforms are able to extend viewing time and make billions in profits.[6]

With this engagement-promoting digital ecosystem in mind, updated research evidence about children's reading and media habits is needed, particularly in developmentally sensitive windows when such habits are established. In this issue of *Pediatrics*, McArthur et al[7] present findings from a large birth cohort in which reading and screen use were assessed at 24, 36, and 60 months of age. The children were born in 2008–2010, so they likely had access to smartphones and tablets.

With three waves of data, the authors were able to statistically control for between-child confounders (eg, family stress) and isolate within-child variation in screen use and reading over time. They found that more screen use at 24 months of age predicted less shared book reading at 36 months of age ($\beta = -.08$), which in turn predicted higher screen use at 60 months of age ($\beta = -.11$).

These results suggest that toddlerhood may be a key window in which children establish preferences for media over reading as a daily activity, which sets the stage for more screen use around kindergarten entry. Daily toddler habits (eg, sleep and feeding) are influenced by the intense emotionality and self-directed behavior that can dominate this period.[8] Therefore, it is possible that toddler demands for media and parents' related low self-efficacy in establishing daily reading routines may drive this association.

Like many large cohort studies, in this study, McArthur et al[7] only assessed one dimension of media use: time. Now that media are engineered to engage young viewers through persuasive enhancements, more longitudinal research is needed that interrogates children's reactions to mobile and interactive design: Are devices coming to bed and meals with them or being grabbed in the moment to calm a tantrum?[9] When young children

Department of Pediatrics, Michigan Medicine, University of Michigan, Ann Arbor, Michigan

Opinions expressed in these commentaries are those of the author and not necessarily those of the American Academy of Pediatrics or its Committees.

DOI: https://doi.org/10.1542/peds.2020-047472

Accepted for publication Mar 19, 2021

Address correspondence to Jenny S. Radesky, MD, Department of Pediatrics, Michigan Medicine, University of Michigan, 300 N Ingalls St, #1107, Ann Arbor, MI 48019. E-mail: jradesky@med.umich.edu

PEDIATRICS (ISSN Numbers: Print, 0031-4005; Online, 1098-4275).

FINANCIAL DISCLOSURE: The author has indicated she has no financial relationships relevant to this article to disclose.

FUNDING: Dr Radesky is supported by a career development award from the National Institute of Child Health and Development (grant K23HD092626). Funded by the National Institutes of Health (NIH).

POTENTIAL CONFLICT OF INTEREST: Dr Radesky receives research funding from Common Sense Media and is a paid consultant of Noggin and Viacom and Melissa & Doug Toys, LLC. None of these products are discussed in this commentary.

COMPANION PAPER: A companion to this article can be found online at www.pediatrics.org/cgi/doi/10.1542/peds.2020-011429.

To cite: Radesky JS. Establishing Early Literacy Habits in a Profit-Driven Digital World. *Pediatrics.* 2021;147(6):e2020047472

COMMENTARY

engage with apps and videos, do they go on "autopilot" and expect to follow a frictionless feed, and how does that influence their more friction-full daily interactions with people and learning? Do they take a "minds-on" orientation to screen media, as they would a book?[5] As the US government debates potentially increasing funding for children and media research (ie, Children and Media Research Advancement Act),[10] these types of questions, and implications for the corporate responsibility of the companies designing children's digital ecosystems, should be prioritized.

REFERENCES

1. High PC, Klass P; Council on Early Childhood. Literacy promotion: an essential component of primary care pediatric practice. *Pediatrics.* 2014; 134(2):404–409
2. Vandewater EA, Bickham DS, Lee JH, Cummings HM, Wartella EA, Rideout VJ. When the television is always on: heavy television exposure and young children's development. *Am Behav Sci.* 2005;48(5):562–577
3. Vandewater EA, Bickham DS, Lee JH. Time well spent? Relating television use to children's free-time activities. *Pediatrics.* 2006;117(2). Available at: www.pediatrics.org/cgi/content/full/117/2/e181
4. Vandewater EA, Bickham DS. The impact of educational television on young children's reading in the context of family stress. *J Appl Dev Psychol.* 2004; 25(6):717–728
5. Meyer M, Zosh JM, McLaren C, et al. How educational are "educational" apps for young children? App store content analysis using the Four Pillars of Learning framework [published online ahead of print February 23, 2021]. *J Child Media.* doi:10.1080/17482798.2021.1882516
6. Statista. Worldwide advertising revenues of YouTube as of 4th quarter 2020. Available at: https://www.statista.com/statistics/289657/youtube-global-quarterly-advertising-revenues/. Accessed March 12, 2021
7. McArthur BA, Browne D, McDonald S, Tough S, Madigan S. Longitudinal associations between screen use and reading in preschool children. *Pediatrics.* 2021;147(6):e2020011429
8. Conway A, Miller AL, Modrek A. Testing reciprocal links between trouble getting to sleep and internalizing behavior problems, and bedtime resistance and externalizing behavior problems in toddlers. *Child Psychiatry Hum Dev.* 2017;48(4):678–689
9. Coyne SM, Shawcroft J, Gale M, et al. Tantrums, toddlers and technology: temperament, media emotion regulation, and problematic media use in early childhood. *Comput Hum Behav.* 2021;120:106762
10. Children and Media Research Advancement Act. HR 1367, 116th Cong, (2019–2020). Available at: https://www.markey.senate.gov/imo/media/doc/CAMRA%20Act.pdf. Accessed March 12, 2021

Differences in Parent-Toddler Interactions With Electronic Versus Print Books

Tiffany G. Munzer, MD,[a] Alison L. Miller, PhD,[b,c] Heidi M. Weeks, PhD,[d] Niko Kaciroti, PhD,[c,e] Jenny Radesky, MD[a]

abstract

OBJECTIVES: Previous research has documented less dialogic interaction between parents and preschoolers during electronic-book reading versus print. Parent-toddler interactions around commercially available tablet-based books have not been described. We examined parent-toddler verbal and nonverbal interactions when reading electronic versus print books.

METHODS: We conducted a videotaped, laboratory-based, counterbalanced study of 37 parent-toddler dyads reading on 3 book formats (enhanced electronic [sound effects and/or animation], basic electronic, and print). We coded verbalizations in 10-second intervals for parents (dialogic, nondialogic, text reading, format related, negative format-related directives, and off task) and children (book related, negative, and off task). Shared positive affect and collaborative book reading were coded on a scale of 1 to 5 (5 = high). Proc Genmod and Proc Mixed analyzed within-subjects variance by book format.

RESULTS: Parents showed significantly more dialogic (print 11.9; enhanced 6.2 [$P < .001$]; basic 8.3 [$P < .001$]), text-reading (print 14.3; enhanced 10.6 [$P = .003$]; basic 14.4 [$P < .001$]), off-task (print 2.3; enhanced 1.3 [$P = .007$]), and total (29.5; enhanced 28.1 [$P = .003$]; basic 29.3 [$P = .005$]) verbalizations with print books and fewer format-related verbalizations (print 1.9; enhanced 10.0 [$P < .001$]; basic 8.3 [$P < .001$]). Toddlers showed more book-related verbalizations (print 15.0; enhanced 11.5 [$P < .001$]; basic 12.5 [$P = .005$]), total verbalizations (print 18.8; enhanced 13.8 [$P < .001$]; basic 15.3 [$P < .001$]), and higher collaboration scores (print 3.1; enhanced 2.7 [$P = .004$]; basic 2.8 [$P = .02$]) with print-book reading.

CONCLUSIONS: Parents and toddlers verbalized less with electronic books, and collaboration was lower. Future studies should examine specific aspects of tablet-book design that support parent-child interaction. Pediatricians may wish to continue promoting shared reading of print books, particularly for toddlers and younger children.

[a]*Department of Pediatrics, Medical School,* [b]*Departments of Health Behavior and Health Education,* [d]*Nutritional Sciences, and* [e]*Biostatistics, School of Public Health, and* [c]*Center for Human Growth and Development, University of Michigan, Ann Arbor, Michigan*

Dr Munzer conceptualized and designed the study, coordinated and supervised data collection, drafted the initial manuscript, and reviewed and revised the manuscript; Dr Miller conceptualized and designed the study and reviewed and revised the manuscript; Dr Weeks conducted the data management, processing, and analyses and reviewed and revised the manuscript; Dr Kaciroti created the data analysis plan, conducted the data analysis, and reviewed and revised the manuscript; Dr Radesky conceptualized and designed the study, coordinated and supervised data collection, and reviewed and revised the manuscript; and all authors approved the final manuscript as submitted and agree to be accountable for all aspects of the work.

DOI: https://doi.org/10.1542/peds.2018-2012

Accepted for publication Dec 10, 2018

WHAT'S KNOWN ON THIS SUBJECT: When preschoolers read electronic books with parents, parents may show less dialogic reading, and talk is often focused on the technology. It is not known whether toddler-parent interactions differ when reading commercially available electronic books compared with print.

WHAT THIS STUDY ADDS: Parents engaged in more dialogic reading with fewer technology-related verbalizations and more parent-toddler verbalizations with print books compared with electronic books. Print books elicited a higher quality of parent-toddler collaborative reading experience compared with electronic books.

To cite: Munzer TG, Miller AL, Weeks HM, et al. Differences in Parent-Toddler Interactions With Electronic Versus Print Books. *Pediatrics.* 2019;143(4):e20182012

ARTICLE

Shared book reading is 1 of the most important developmental activities parents can engage in with their children.[1] Shared book reading exposes children to more sophisticated speech and knowledge,[2,3] and provides unhurried time to build attachment,[2,4] in turn promoting executive functioning skills.[5] Nonverbal interactions during shared book reading, such as parental warmth and child enthusiasm, foster interest in reading and are associated with improved literacy later in life.[6,7] In particular, parent dialogic reading practices (comments and questions that go beyond the written word and connect the story to child experiences) are believed to promote child expressive language, engagement, and literacy.[8–10]

With rapid increases in electronic-book and mobile-device ownership,[11,12] a growing amount of children's reading is taking place electronically on electronic readers or tablets. However, pediatricians are unsure whether to promote their use because previous studies suggest both benefits and drawbacks to electronic reading for preschoolers and older children.[13,14] Previous literature has shown that electronic books may facilitate engagement, particularly among reluctant preschoolers and kindergarteners who are learning to read.[14–16] Certain embedded tools, such as dictionaries, may improve vocabulary and story comprehension in kindergarteners.[15,17,18] However, preschoolers and kindergarteners also reproduced fewer narrative details[19] and sequenced story events with lower accuracy after reading enhanced electronic books compared with print books.[13,20] Lower comprehension during electronic-book reading may be due to less adult verbal elaboration[14] and scaffolding[16] and extraneous "hot-spot" enhancements, which may distract from story content.[17] Yet, adult verbal elaboration and parental scaffolding is crucial for young children's learning,[21] particularly regarding digital media.[22–24]

An existing gap in knowledge is how toddlers and parents interact around electronic books. Developmentally, toddlerhood (~24–36 months old) is characterized by emerging language and social-emotional skills as well as immature executive functioning skills. These developmental differences may make toddlers particularly susceptible to the distractions[25] in enhanced electronic books. Additionally, because of their immature memory flexibility, toddlers depend more on adult scaffolding to transfer information from digital media to the real world,[26,27] have more difficulty learning information presented in digital media compared with in-person interactions,[23] and retain information better when digital media are viewed with an adult.[24] Only 1 electronic-book study has been conducted in toddlers, finding that toddlers remembered a novel word better on an electronic book compared with print, but parents read the text and pointed more when interacting over print.[27] This study used an electronic book without digital enhancements that was not commercially available; therefore, results do not generalize to tablet-based books available to families.[22] To our knowledge, no studies have examined dialogic and nonverbal interactions between parents and toddlers when reading electronic books.

For pediatric providers to make informed decisions about recommending electronic books, more needs to be known about differences in parent-child interactions during these types of reading encounters with toddlers, a developmental range that is underrepresented in current literature. In this study, we aim to address these gaps by examining the frequency of parent verbalizations that are important to early language and literacy (eg, dialogic reading), child verbalizations, and quality of the shared book-reading experience during the reading of commercially available electronic and print books.

METHODS

Study Design

We conducted an experimental, laboratory-based study consisting of a video-recorded free play, book-reading protocol, and surveys lasting ~75 minutes. Toddler-parent dyads were assigned to 1 of 36 counterbalanced book-format orders. Parents were compensated $50 for participating. The University of Michigan Institutional Review Board approved this study.

Participants

We recruited 37 parent-toddler dyads from the University of Michigan online research registry (UMhealthresearch.org) and community-based settings, including pediatric offices, child care centers, and community centers. To not bias recruitment toward parents with particular digital media views, language stated generically that the study involved coming to the University of Michigan, where "you and your child would be videotaped while playing with toys and books." Parents contacted researchers via the research registry, e-mail, or phone and underwent phone-based screening. Inclusion criteria were as follows: (1) child age 24 to 36 months, (2) child did not have a developmental delay or serious medical condition, (3) parent read English sufficiently to complete questionnaires and consent, (4) parent was a legal and/or physical custodial guardian, and (5) parent and child did not have uncorrected hearing or vision impairments.

Procedure

At the study visit, parents provided written informed consent. The laboratory room was set up to approximate a living room and contained a 1-way mirror, couches, 3 books in boxes (2 tablet books and 1 print book), and video cameras.

Participants first completed a 5-minute, video-recorded free play with nondigital toys. They then completed a random, preassigned reading activity with an enhanced electronic book, a basic electronic book, and a print book occurring in counterbalanced order (Fig 1). Figure 2 includes 1 example permutation. Books were placed in open boxes labeled 1 to 3 out of children's reach. Parents received instructions to start with the book in box 1, that they have "5 minutes to look at it," and to complete books sequentially as prompted.

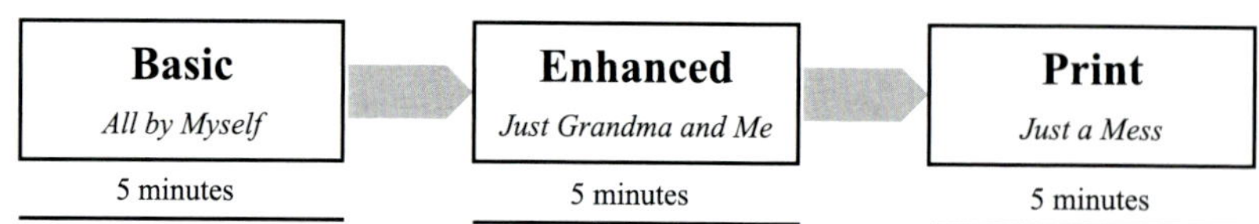

FIGURE 2

Sample of 1 book-reading permutation completed by a participant.

Book Formats

Three Mercer Mayer "Little Critter" books (*Just Grandma and Me*, *All by Myself*, and *Just a Mess*) were chosen because of their similar length, reading difficulty, and availability in all 3 formats. Print books were 8×8-inch softcovers. Basic electronic-book capabilities allowed for swiping to turn the pages and tapping illustrations to elicit the appearance of words but without autonarration or additional features, such as sound effects. Enhanced electronic books contained audiovisual hot spots: tapping illustrations would result in the appearance and narration of the word (eg, tapping a seagull picture resulted in the appearance and narration of the word "seagull") coupled with sound effects. Tapping other pictures or turning a page produced a sound effect (eg, tapping a dog would produce the sound of a dog panting, and turning the page to a beach produced sounds of ocean waves). Although autonarration of the story was disabled on both electronic-book formats, tapping and holding down an individual sentence in the enhanced electronic book would narrate that text, but this feature was only briefly used by 2 dyads. Basic and enhanced electronic books were preloaded on a 10-inch Samsung Galaxy tablet computer, which contained no other applications. Parents received instruction to select "read it myself" such that the electronic book was not narrating the book text.

Survey Measures

Parents completed surveys regarding covariates for potential inclusion in statistical models, including demographic information (parent age, sex, educational attainment, household income, race and/or ethnicity, relationship to child, and marital status; child's age, sex, ethnicity, and prematurity) and standardized measures of child language, social-emotional development, and digital media–use practices.

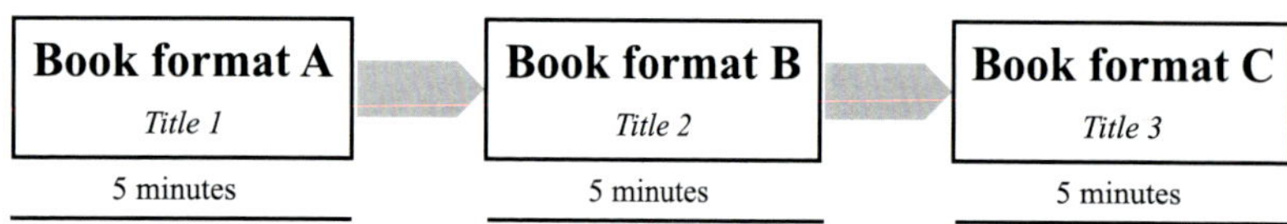

FIGURE 1

Reading protocol. The reading protocol consisted of a preassigned sequential reading activity of an enhanced electronic book, a basic electronic book, and a print book occurring in a counterbalanced fashion in 1 of 6 book-format permutations: (1) enhanced, basic, print; (2) enhanced, print, basic; (3) basic, enhanced, print; (4) basic, print, enhanced; (5) print, basic, enhanced; or (6) print, enhanced, basic. Within each book-format permutation, the order of 3 different book titles was counter-balanced, achieving a total of 36 unique permutations. Thus, all participants read the same 3 books, but not all books were read in the same format or order across participants.

The MacArthur-Bates Communicative Developmental Inventory (CDI) short form assessed toddler language development. This 100-word validated[28] and reliable[29] vocabulary checklist generated a percentile score from total words produced and accounted for age.[24]

The Brief Infant-Toddler Social and Emotional Assessment (BITSEA) is a validated[30] and reliable[25] 42-item questionnaire that screens for child social-emotional problems. Parents rated items on a 3-point Likert scale generating the Problem and Competence subscales (Cronbach α = 0.68 and 0.58, respectively).

Standardized questions assessed the frequency of home child digital media use (including tablet, smartphone, and electronic-book usage) and parental mediation strategies (instructive, restrictive, and coviewing).[31]

Coding Parent-Toddler Verbal Interactions

We developed a verbal coding scheme based on previous literature on dialogic reading[8] and shared electronic-book reading.[14] For each 10-second interval, researchers coded 1 for a specific verbalization occurring or 0 for not occurring; interval verbalization counts were summed within each 5-minute book condition. Verbalization categories were not mutually exclusive; parents and children could have >1 type per 10-second interval, although each sentence was only coded in 1 category. Please see the coding definitions in Tables 1 and 2 for

TABLE 1 Coding Definitions and Examples of Parent Verbalizations

	Definition	Examples	Cohen's κ
Dialogic	Dialogic reading techniques often prompt a child to expand and elaborate on concepts related to the story. These were defined as follows: parent asks open-ended question, expands on an idea the child has, repeats what the child says, or relates the story content to the child's experience.	"What's happening here?" "What did they do next?" "What did you think about that book?" "Remember when you went to the beach with Dad?" Child says, "Here is a wagon," and parent replies, "a big, red wagon."	0.77
Nondialogic	Nondialogic reading techniques were related to story content but have not been previously shown to elicit the same quantity of child verbalizations as dialogic verbalizations. These were defined as follows: parent labels something, asks a simple question requiring only a name or label, makes a pointing request of the child, makes an attention prompt, or talks about the process of reading.	"What is that?" "Show me the cat." "Look at this!" "There's Grandma!"	0.74
Text read	Parent reads directly from the book text.	"We went to the beach, just grandma and me."	0.86
Format related	These are verbalizations that are related to the book format. Parent comments on, asks a question about, or adds a directive regarding an aspect of the print or tablet interface.	"Great job, you're turning the page!" "Can I hold the book or tablet?" "Go ahead and turn the page." "You can push the button here." "Swipe with your finger."	0.84
Negative format-related directives	Parent makes a negative directive that is related to the book format. For instance, the parent tells the child not to do something related to how the book or tablet functions.	"You can't keep pressing the back button." "Don't turn the page." "Don't rip the book." "Don't turn the volume up." "Don't touch that button."	0.80
Off task	These are unrelated to the book content or book format and include all other parent verbalizations that are not categorized as above.	"You can have your goldfish later." "We are going to the store after this."	0.79

parent and child verbalizations. Parent and child utterances were independently summed to calculate total verbalizations. Undergraduate students blinded to the hypothesis coded to reliability with Cohen's κ of at least 0.70.

Coding Parent-Toddler Nonverbal Interactions

We developed 2 global coding schemes based on existing literature on shared print-book reading to assess parent-toddler nonverbal interactions: shared positive affect[32] and collaborative book-reading experience.[33–35] Codes were applied on the basis of the full 5 minutes per book condition on a scale of 1 to 5 (Table 3). The 5-minute free-play session was also coded for shared positive affect and examined as a potential covariate representing baseline parent-child interaction quality.

Analysis

We conducted Poisson regressions using Proc Genmod to compare each verbal outcome by book format, adjusting for total elapsed time, given the occasional variation in reading duration. Proc Mixed was used to compare differences in positive affect and collaborative book reading by book format. All models included a repeated measures statement to allow for within-subjects comparison of verbal and nonverbal outcomes by book-format condition. Although the counterbalanced design accounted for between-subjects variance in factors known to influence book-reading behaviors, such as sociodemographic characteristics, we included covariates in final models with $P < .05$ to improve model fit (eg, order of book presentation, parent income, race and/or ethnicity, child sex, CDI or BITSEA score, and home media practices). A sensitivity

TABLE 2 Coding Definitions and Examples of Child Verbalizations

	Definition	Examples	Cohen's κ
Book related	Child labels a picture, answers a parent question, repeats what the parent is saying, or talks about a function of the book.	"I want to read this." "I press the button." "Look, a spider!"	0.81
Negative	Child says no or makes a comment in a defiant or negative manner.	"No, Daddy, I do it." "I hold it."	0.71
Other	These are verbalizations that do not fall into the above categories. Unintelligible utterances that are not clearly related to the book were also included.	"Can I have water?" "I want to go home."	0.72

TABLE 3 Nonverbal Coding Definitions

Definition	Shared Positive Affect Quantity of shared enjoyment between dyad	Collaborative Book Reading Quality of shared reading experience
Intraclass correlation	0.84	0.75
Code 1	A score of 1 was marked by little positive shared affect or enjoyment, several instances of negative affect that occur more frequently than instances of positive affect, and/or the child having a tantrum or refusal of prolonged duration or high frequency.	A score of 1 was marked by greater distance between the parent and child, the parent making few attempts to engage the child or being overly directive and/or intrusive, or the child missing social bids from the parent or being confrontational and/or defiant.
Code 3	A score of 3 was marked by small-to-moderate amounts of positive affect between the dyad with brief but unsustained instances of negative affect, or the dyad may be primarily affectively neutral.	A score of 3 was marked by some instances of close dyad proximity with some instances of greater distance between them, some attempts of parent-child engagement but less in frequency than a code 4 or 5, and/or the dyad seeming more focused on the reading task than on each other.
Code 5	A score of 5 was marked by frequent displays of shared positive affect with the dyad showing definite pleasure with each other (eg, high frequency of smiling, laughing, praise, and warmth).	A score of 5 was marked by the dyad being comfortably nestled together with a shared view of the book, a highly responsive parent, and an actively engaged child who exhibits minimal defiance.

analysis excluding 1 participant who cried during the entirety of 1 book-reading condition did not reveal differences; therefore, all participants were included. All analyses were completed in SAS 9.4 (SAS Institute, Inc, Cary, NC).

RESULTS

As shown in Table 4, children were 29.2 months old, and parents were 33.5 years old. Of the parents, 81% were mothers, 76% had a 4-year college degree or more, and 89% were married. Of the children, 54% were boys, 57% were non-Hispanic white, 16% were non-Hispanic African American, and 27% were of other race and/or ethnicity.

Figure 3 shows the number of intervals containing each type of parent verbalization. Parent dialogic verbalizations were greater with print (11.9 intervals [SE = 1.1]) versus either enhanced electronic (6.2 intervals [SE = 0.7]; $P < .001$) or basic electronic books (8.3 intervals [SE = 0.9]; $P < .001$). Parent nondialogic verbalizations were greater with print (17.7 [SE = 0.7]) versus basic electronic books (15.7 [SE = 0.8]; $P = .008$). Parents read the book text more with print (14.3 [SE = 1.0]; $P = .003$) or basic electronic (14.4 [SE = 1.1]; $P < .001$) compared with enhanced electronic books (10.6 [SE = 0.9]). Parents made fewer format-related and negative format-related directives when engaging over print books versus enhanced or basic electronic books (Fig 3). Parents had

TABLE 4 Participant Characteristics ($N = 37$)

Sample	Result
Child age, mo, mean (SD)	29.2 (4.2)
Parent age, y, mean (SD)	33.5 (4.0)
Parent relationship to child, *n* (%)	
Mother	30 (81)
Father	7 (19)
Child sex, *n* (%)	
Boys	20 (54)
Girls	17 (46)
Child race and/or ethnicity, *n* (%)	
White, non-Hispanic	21 (57)
African American, non-Hispanic	6 (16)
Hispanic or other	10 (27)
Parent education, *n* (%)	
Some college courses	4 (11)
2-y college degree	5 (13)
4-y college degree	14 (38)
More than 4-y college degree	14 (38)
Parent marital status, *n* (%)	
Single	4 (11)
Married	33 (89)
Child has used tablet to read a book, *n* (%)	
Almost never	23 (62)
Rarely	2 (5)
Occasionally	4 (11)
Often	6 (16)
Most of the time	2 (5)
Daily time spent reading books together, *n* (%)	
Not used	8 (22)
<30 min	16 (43)
30 min–1 h	9 (24)
1–2 h	3 (8)
3–4 h	1 (3)
CDI percentile, mean (SD)	52.9 (33.4)
BITSEA Problem subscale, mean (SD)	6.7 (3.8)
BITSEA Competence subscale, mean (SD)	19.1 (2.2)

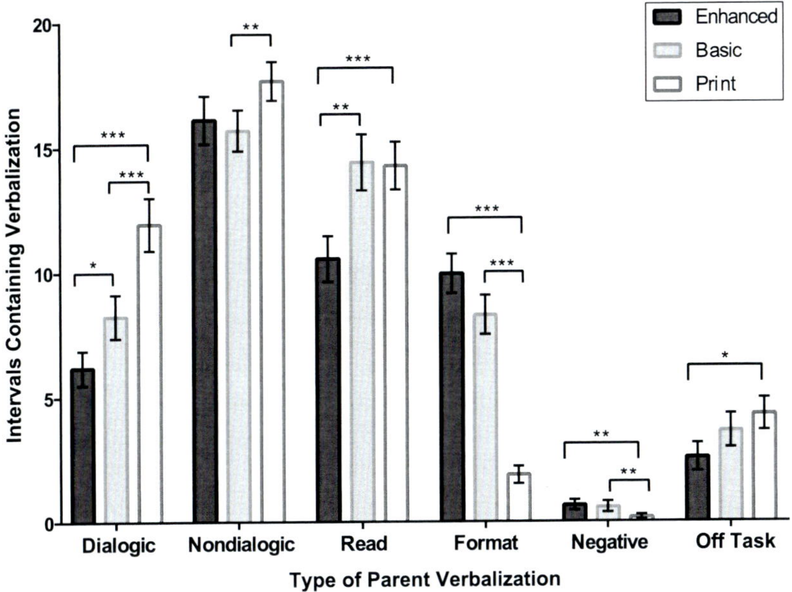

FIGURE 3
Adjusted means for the presence of parent verbalizations occurring with enhanced electronic, basic electronic, and print books. * $P < .05$; ** $P < .01$; *** $P < .001$.

more total verbalizations when interacting over print books (29.5 [SE = 0.2]) versus enhanced electronic books (28.1 [SE = 0.4]; $P = .003$) and more so over basic electronic books (29.3 [SE = 0.3]; $P = .005$) versus enhanced electronic books.

Figure 4 includes the number of intervals containing each type of toddler verbalization. Toddlers' book-content verbalizations were greater with print (15.0 [SE = 1.2]) versus either enhanced electronic (11.5 [SE = 0.9]; $P < .001$) or basic electronic books (12.5 [SE = 1.1]; $P = .005$). Toddlers had no differences in negative verbalizations across all formats but had more off-task verbalizations with print (2.3 [SE = 0.3]) versus enhanced electronic books (1.3 [SE = 0.3]; $P = .007$). Total toddler verbalizations were greater with print (18.8 [SE = 1.1]) versus either enhanced electronic (13.8 [SE = 0.9]; $P < .001$) or basic electronic books (15.3 [SE = 1.0]; $P < .001$).

Figure 5 includes nonverbal outcomes by book format. Shared positive affect was similar across all book formats. Dyads' collaborative book-reading scores were higher with print (3.1 [SE = 0.2]) versus either enhanced electronic (2.7 [SE = 0.2]; $P = .004$) or basic electronic books (2.8 [SE = 0.2]; $P = .02$).

DISCUSSION

Developmental benefits of shared book reading have been attributed to the quality of parent-child interactions occurring around books, particularly in prereaders such as toddlers, who rely heavily on parents to understand story content.[8] These interactions include the quantity of words spoken, how parents tailor content to children's experiences to support learning, and asking open-ended questions to promote child expressive language.[5,8] Our findings suggest that high-quality dialogic practices are less common, and parents and toddlers speak less overall and in a less collaborative manner, when reading electronic books compared with print. Parents read the text less in enhanced electronic books, making more format-related comments and negative directives when reading electronic books.

Similar to previous studies in preschoolers,[17] we found that electronic-book enhancements were likely interfering with parents' ability to engage in dialogic reading. Dialogic, parent-guided conversation promotes toddler expressive-language development and supports preliteracy skills, which are crucial for independent reading,[8] far more than reading only text or making simple (nondialogic) comments, although these are also important.[1] Parents strengthen their children's ability to acquire knowledge by relating new content to their children's lived experiences.[21,36] There is a large body of literature showing that this type of adult scaffolding is especially important for toddlers to transfer information from digital media to the real world because toddlers in particular learn and retain novel information better from in-person interactions than from digital media.[22–24,26,27,37] However, such practices occurred less frequently with electronic books, which raises the question of whether electronic books have lower educational potential for toddlers.

Parents also asked fewer simple questions, commented about the storyline less, and read less during electronic-book conditions compared with print. These behaviors are important because they promote child receptive language by exposing children to novel vocabulary and more complex syntax than conversations occurring during daily activities.[1]

Even interactions over basic electronic books contained fewer dialogic and total parent verbalizations compared with print, suggesting that affordances of the tablet (and not only the interactive design) may be influencing parents' behavior. Parents and children may conceptualize tablets as being

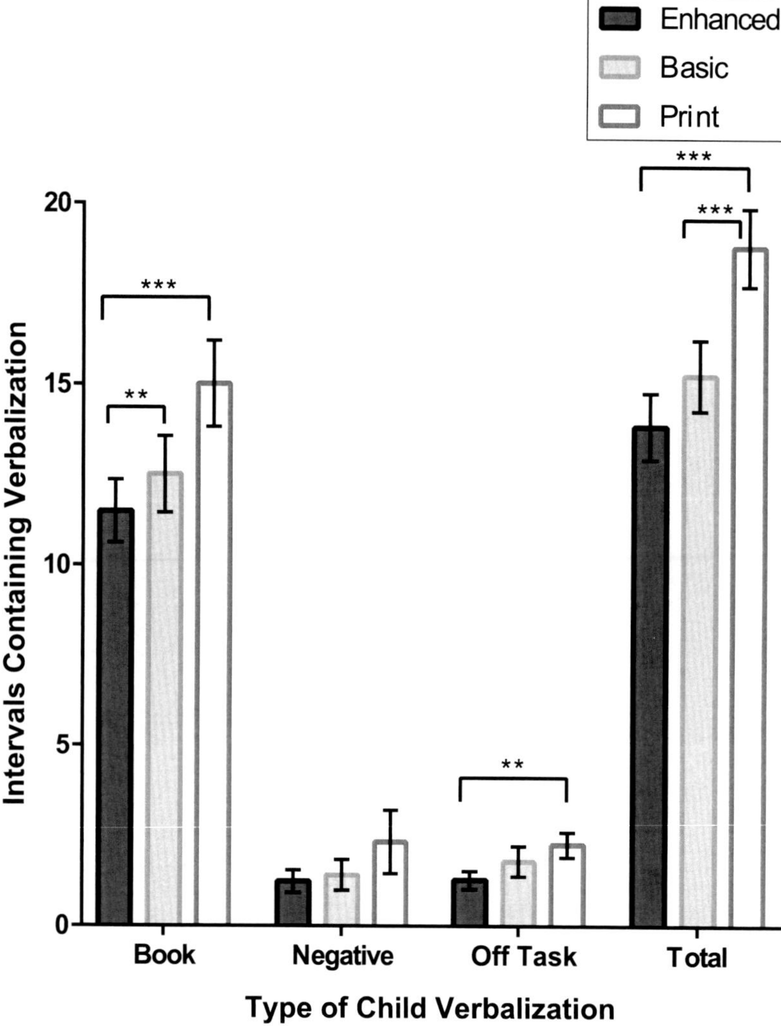

FIGURE 4
Adjusted means for the presence of toddler verbalizations occurring with enhanced electronic, basic electronic, and print books. * $P < .05$; ** $P < .01$; *** $P < .001$.

individually used rather than shared objects. Indeed, 1 study revealed that children tend to create solitary spaces when engaging in tablet play compared with traditional toy play, leaving less space for their parents to coview and ignoring parent bids for attention.[38] Similarly, parents reported a sense of pride and relief when their children independently engaged with a tablet device without help,[39] and we acknowledge that this independence may be perceived as a potential benefit of electronic books. We hypothesize that the tablet itself may reduce opportunities for parent-child interactions during book reading.

Children changed their behavior as a function of book format, verbalizing more when reading the print book. This finding may be related to greater parent dialogic reading with print books versus electronic books, which provides positive reinforcement for toddler speech. Children's tendency to become occupied in repeated tapping or swiping on electronic books may also have supplanted speech production. Repetitive tapping and swiping may not constitute sufficient engagement to learn new concepts because it is thought to represent cause-and-effect play rather than "minds-on" activity.[21] True meaningful engagement (active involvement occurring in a rich social context without distractions) fosters the most effective learning from media.[21] Previous research in preschoolers supports this concept because distracting digital enhancements interfere with parent scaffolding, which leads to reduced child story comprehension and fewer child verbalizations.[13,14] Opportunities to practice expressive language, such as those occurring with print books, are important because early language skills strongly predict future linguistic and cognitive aptitude in school.[40]

The high frequency of format-related verbalizations (eg, directing the child to turn the page) observed during both electronic-book conditions may displace book-related verbal exchanges that dyads engaged in with print books. This is consistent with previous research: although parents showed the same number of verbal exchanges with preschoolers around electronic versus print books, exchanges tended to be related to technology rather than story content.[14] It is possible that parents made more format-related verbalizations to orient their children to a new experience because electronic books were novel to 62% of the children in this sample; however, 79% had previously played with tablets and/or mobile devices. The negative and directive nature of parent format-related verbalizations may indicate a need for more behavioral management with electronic books compared with print.

Parents and children had more off-task verbalizations with the print book versus electronic book, which is similar to previous studies in preschoolers.[14] This could be related to persuasive tablet-design features, which may command parent and

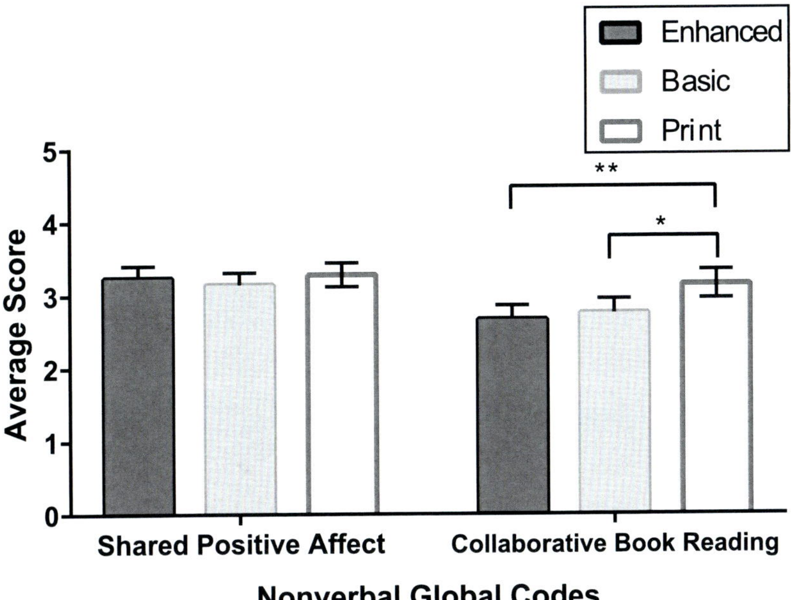

FIGURE 5
Adjusted means (5 = high) for dyad social-emotional outcomes occurring with enhanced electronic, basic electronic, and print books. * $P < .05$; ** $P < .01$.

child attention, at the expense of attending to one another, an effect that is known to occur with traditional screen media, such as television.[41–43] It is challenging to discern whether this attentional focus resulted in improved learning because toddler reading comprehension is difficult to assess. However, as mentioned above, toddlers may be engaged in ways that may be less educationally enriching when reading electronic compared with print books.

Our study was the first to examine nonverbal aspects of electronic-book reading in toddlers both through shared positive affect and collaborative book reading. These nonverbal behaviors during reading are important because they foster a love of reading[7] and promote secure parent-child attachment,[1] which has been implicated in resilience,[44] physical health,[45] and quality of future relationships.[46] Comparable to previous studies in preschoolers,[14] dyads with high shared positive affect consistently showed this across all formats, suggesting that electronic books may be equally enjoyable for dyads despite other limitations. The quality of collaborative reading was likely lower for electronic books because observationally, parents and toddlers frequently sat separately, could not easily view the book, or appeared to struggle for tablet possession. These behaviors during tablet-based play are documented in recent work[38] and merit further study. Our results may explain previous findings that parents report preferring shared reading over print versus electronic books with toddlers.[47]

Limitations include the small sample size from 1 geographic area, the use of only 1 type of book-reading application (which limits generalizability), and that the age range of our study sample precluded assessment of reading comprehension.[48] Strengths include experimental methodology, the use of commercially available books available in 3 formats, a diverse sample, and the within-subjects design, which allowed for direct comparison of the reading experience within each dyad. Future studies should consider other facets of nonverbal interactions or moderating effects of dyad characteristics, such as parent literacy level, child temperament, or home media-use practices. Replication of this study by using different applications (this application had a particular set of enhancements) in other contexts, such as home or school settings, is necessary. Although parent-child interactions are critical for toddler learning, directly examining toddler learning from print versus electronic books is another important area for future work.

CONCLUSIONS

Given the decreased quantity of parent-child verbalizations and quality of interactions occurring with the electronic books that we studied, pediatricians may wish to recommend print books over electronic books with distracting features for parent-toddler shared reading. In considering affordances of electronic books that promote learning, software designers should limit irrelevant audiovisual enhancements for toddlers. Parents reading electronic books with toddlers should consider engaging as they would with print and minimize focus on elements of the technology itself.

ACKNOWLEDGMENTS

We thank Rosa Ball, Ranya Alkhayyat, Joy Boakye, and Anastasia Pacifico for their diligent and wonderful work on this study.

ABBREVIATIONS

BITSEA: Brief Infant-Toddler Social and Emotional Assessment
CDI: Communicative Developmental Inventory

Address correspondence to Tiffany G. Munzer, MD, Department of Pediatrics, University of Michigan Medical School, 300 N. Ingalls St, 1024 NW, Ann Arbor, MI 48109-5406. E-mail: chungti@med.umich.edu

PEDIATRICS (ISSN Numbers: Print, 0031-4005; Online, 1098-4275).

FINANCIAL DISCLOSURE: Dr Radesky is paid to write articles for PBS Parents and is on the board of directors and consults for Melissa and Doug; the other authors have indicated they have no financial relationships relevant to this article to disclose.

FUNDING: Funded by the 2017 Academic Pediatric Association Reach Out and Read Young Investigator Award (principal investigator: Dr Radesky), which made it possible to conceptualize, implement, collect, and analyze data and write this article, and supported by the *Eunice Kennedy Shriver* National Institute of Child Health and Human Development (grant 5T32HD079350-02), which made it possible to conceptualize and write this article. Funded by the National Institutes of Health (NIH).

POTENTIAL CONFLICT OF INTEREST: Dr Radesky is paid to write articles for PBS Parents and is on the board of directors and consults for Melissa and Doug; the other authors have indicated they have no potential conflicts of interest to disclose.

REFERENCES

1. Zuckerman B. Promoting early literacy in pediatric practice: twenty years of reach out and read. *Pediatrics*. 2009; 124(6):1660–1665
2. Isbell R, Sobol J, Lindauer L, Lowrance A. The effects of storytelling and story reading on the oral language complexity and story comprehension of young children. *Early Child Educ J*. 2004; 32(3):157–163
3. Deckner DF, Adamson LB, Bakeman R. Child and maternal contributions to shared reading: effects on language and literacy development. *J Appl Dev Psychol*. 2006;27(1):31–41
4. Xie QW, Chan CHY, Ji Q, Chan CLW. Psychosocial effects of parent-child book reading interventions: a meta-analysis. *Pediatrics*. 2018;141(4): e20172675
5. Mendelsohn AL, Cates CB, Weisleder A, et al. Reading aloud, play, and social-emotional development. *Pediatrics*. 2018;141(5):e20173393
6. Baker L, Mackler K, Sonnenschein S, Serpell R. Parents' interactions with their first-grade children during storybook reading and relations with subsequent home reading activity and reading achievement. *J Sch Psychol*. 2001;39(5):415–438
7. Kassow DZ. Parent-child shared book reading: quality versus quantity of reading interactions between parents and young children. *Talaris Research Institute*. 2006;1(1):1–9
8. Whitehurst GJ, Arnold DS, Epstein JN, Angell AL, Smith M, Fischel JE. A picture book reading intervention in day care and home for children from low-income families. *Dev Psychol*. 1994;30(5): 679–689
9. Arnold DS, Whitehurst GJ. Accelerating language development through picture book reading: A summary of dialogic reading and its effect. In: Dickinson DK, ed. *Bridges to Literacy: Children, Families, and Schools*. Hoboken, NJ: Wiley-Blackwell; 1994:103–128
10. Lever R, Sénéchal M. Discussing stories: on how a dialogic reading intervention improves kindergartners' oral narrative construction. *J Exp Child Psychol*. 2011; 108(1):1–24
11. Perrin A. *Book Reading 2016*. Washington, DC: Pew Research Center; 2016
12. Kabali HK, Irigoyen MM, Nunez-Davis R, et al. Exposure and use of mobile media devices by young children. *Pediatrics*. 2015;136(6):1044–1050
13. Krcmar M, Cingel DP. Parent–child joint reading in traditional and electronic formats. *Media Psychol*. 2014;17(3): 262–281
14. Chiong C, Ree J, Takeuchi L, Erickson I. *Comparing Parent-Child Co-Reading on Print, Basic, and Enhanced E-Book Platforms: A Cooney Center Quick Report*. New York City, NY: The Joan Ganz Cooney Center; 2012
15. Korat O, Shamir A, Arbiv L. E-books as support for emergent writing with and without adult assistance. *Educ Inf Technol*. 2011;16(3):301–318
16. Lauricella AR, Barr R, Calvert SL. Parent–child interactions during traditional and computer storybook reading for children's comprehension: implications for electronic storybook design. *Int J Child Comput Interact*. 2014;2(1):17–25
17. Bus AG, Takacs ZK, Kegel CA. Affordances and limitations of electronic storybooks for young children's emergent literacy. *Dev Rev*. 2015;35:79–97
18. Lewin C. Exploring the effects of talking book software in UK primary classrooms. *J Res Read*. 2000;23(2): 149–157
19. De Jong MT, Bus AG. Quality of book-reading matters for emergent readers: an experiment with the same book in a regular or electronic format. *J Educ Psychol*. 2002;94(1):145
20. Parish-Morris J, Mahajan N, Hirsh-Pasek K, Golinkoff RM, Collins MF. Once upon a time: parent–child dialogue and storybook reading in the electronic era. *Mind Brain Educ*. 2013;7(3):200–211
21. Vygotsky L. Zone of proximal development. In: Cole M, ed. *Mind in Society: The Development of Higher Psychological Processes*. Cambridge, MA: Harvard University Press; 1987:157
22. Strouse GA, Ganea PA. Toddlers' word learning and transfer from electronic and print books. *J Exp Child Psychol*. 2017;156:129–142
23. Krcmar M, Grela B, Lin K. Can toddlers learn vocabulary from television? An experimental approach. *Media Psychol*. 2007;10(1):41–63
24. Sims C, Colunga E. Parent-child screen media co-viewing: influences on toddlers' word learning and retention.

Paper presented at: *Proceedings of the Annual Meeting of the Cognitive Science Society*; August 1–3, 2013; Montreal, QC

25. Welsh MC, Pennington BF, Groisser DB. A normative-developmental study of executive function: a window on prefrontal function in children. *Dev Neuropsychol*. 1991;7(2):131–149
26. Strouse GA, Troseth GL, O'Doherty KD, Saylor MM. Co-viewing supports toddlers' word learning from contingent and noncontingent video. *J Exp Child Psychol*. 2018;166:310–326
27. Barr R. Memory constraints on infant learning from picture books, television, and touchscreens. *Child Dev Perspect*. 2013;7(4):205–210
28. Dale PS. The validity of a parent report measure of vocabulary and syntax at 24 months. *J Speech Hear Res*. 1991;34(3): 565–571
29. Nordahl-Hansen A, Kaale A, Ulvund S. Inter-rater reliability of parent and preschool teacher ratings of language in children with autism. *Res Autism Spectr Disord*. 2013;7(11):1391–1396
30. Karabekiroglu K, Briggs-Gowan MJ, Carter AS, Rodopman-Arman A, Akbas S. The clinical validity and reliability of the Brief Infant-Toddler Social and Emotional Assessment (BITSEA). *Infant Behav Dev*. 2010;33(4):503–509
31. Valkenburg PM, Krcmar M, Peeters AL, Marseille NM. Developing a scale to assess three styles of television mediation: "instructive mediation," "restrictive mediation," and "social coviewing". *J Broadcast Electron Media*. 1999;43(1):52–66
32. Frosch CA, Cox MJ, Goldman BD. Infant-parent attachment and parental and child behavior during parent-toddler storybook interaction. *Merrill-Palmer Q*. 2001;47(4):445–474
33. Eyberg SM, Robinson EA. *Dyadic Parent-Child Interaction Coding System*. Seattle, WA: Parenting Clinic, University of Washington; 1981
34. Rocissano L, Slade A, Lynch V. Dyadic synchrony and toddler compliance. *Dev Psychol*. 1987;23(5):698
35. Sonnenschein S, Munsterman K. The influence of home-based reading interactions on 5-year-olds' reading motivations and early literacy development. *Early Child Res Q*. 2002; 17(3):318–337
36. Wadsworth BJ. *Piaget's Theory of Cognitive and Affective Development: Foundations of Constructivism*. White Plains, NY: Longman Publishing; 1996
37. Reiser RA, Tessmer MA, Phelps PC. Adult-child interaction in children's learning from "Sesame Street". *ECTJ*. 1984;32(4):217–223
38. Hiniker A, Lee B, Kientz JA, Radesky JS. Let's play!: digital and analog play between preschoolers and parents. In: *Proceedings of the 2018 CHI Conference on Human Factors in Computing Systems*; April 21–26, 2018; Montreal, QC
39. Radesky JS, Eisenberg S, Kistin CJ, et al. Overstimulated consumers or next-generation learners? Parent tensions about child mobile technology use. *Ann Fam Med*. 2016;14(6):503–508
40. Marchman VA, Fernald A. Speed of word recognition and vocabulary knowledge in infancy predict cognitive and language outcomes in later childhood. *Dev Sci*. 2008;11(3):F9–F16
41. Kirkorian HL, Pempek TA, Murphy LA, Schmidt ME, Anderson DR. The impact of background television on parent-child interaction. *Child Dev*. 2009;80(5): 1350–1359
42. Pempek TA, Kirkorian HL, Anderson DR. The effects of background television on the quantity and quality of child-directed speech by parents. *J Child Media*. 2014;8(3):211–222
43. Schmidt ME, Pempek TA, Kirkorian HL, Lund AF, Anderson DR. The effects of background television on the toy play behavior of very young children. *Child Dev*. 2008;79(4):1137–1151
44. Mikulincer M, Florian V. The relationship between adult attachment styles and emotional and cognitive reactions to stressful events. In: Simpson JA, Rholes WS, eds. *Attachement Theory and Close Relationships*. New York: Guilford Press; 1998:143–165
45. Puig J, Englund MM, Simpson JA, Collins WA. Predicting adult physical illness from infant attachment: a prospective longitudinal study. *Health Psychol*. 2013; 32(4):409–417
46. Brennan KA, Shaver PR. Dimensions of adult attachment, affect regulation, and romantic relationship functioning. *Pers Soc Psychol Bull*. 1995;21(3):267–283
47. Strouse GA, Ganea PA. Parent-toddler behavior and language differ when reading electronic and print picture books. *Front Psychol*. 2017;8:677
48. Keenan JM, Betjemann RS, Olson RK. Reading comprehension tests vary in the skills they assess: differential dependence on decoding and oral comprehension. *Sci Stud Read*. 2008; 12(3):281–300

Electronic Children's Books: Promises Not Yet Fulfilled

Suzy Tomopoulos, MD, Perri Klass, MD, Alan L. Mendelsohn, MD

The infant-toddler period is increasingly recognized as crucial for early brain and child development and school readiness.[1] Parents can support cognitive, language, and social-emotional development during this period through positive parenting activities, such as reading aloud and playing together. Although parents are inundated with information suggesting that new technology can enhance or even replace books to enhance child development, little is known about whether this is true, especially in early childhood.

In this issue of *Pediatrics*, Munzer et al[2] have sought to narrow the data gap by studying interactions that take place when parents and children engage using electronic children's books. Ideally, electronic books could increase access to a range of children's literature through adaptation to ubiquitous digital platforms, such as tablets and electronic readers, and by offering books in multiple languages. They could make developmentally and culturally appropriate reading materials easily accessible at low cost to low-income families in the United States and globally. However, it could also be that tablet-based interfaces are less effective at supporting beneficial interactions than reading print books, especially if features, such as touch activation, are distracting.

One reason books and toys are so important is that they can act as props to support interactions that foster early child development.[3,4] Maintaining conversation with an infant or toddler is not easy, and shared book reading supports more verbal interaction than any other activity.[5] An example is the back and forth of "dialogic reading,"[6,7] in which parents expand on text based on the child's interests and place the content and narrative of the book in context. Also, reading print books creates an opportunity for a special time not built around any screen or device in a way that supports the parent-child relationship and relational health more broadly.[8] Taken together, shared book reading with print books promotes cognitive, language, early literacy, and social-emotional development that strongly support children's successful transition to school and subsequent learning and achievement.

Can current electronic books function similarly to print books in scaffolding interactions that are critical for early child development and school readiness? To address this question, the authors used an experimental design, in which parents of 37 2- to 3-year-olds were asked to read print books, basic electronic books, and electronic books with enhanced features in randomized order. Analyses revealed increased beneficial interactions with print books, including more dialogic reading, text reading, and child engagement in content, compared with either type of electronic book and evidence of barriers to positive interactions (indicated by distracting comments related to the book format and struggles over tablet possession), especially for electronic books with enhanced features.

Department of Pediatrics, School of Medicine, New York University, New York, New York

DOI: https://doi.org/10.1542/peds.2019-0191

Accepted for publication Jan 25, 2019

Address correspondence to Suzy Tomopoulos, MD, Department of Pediatrics, NYU School of Medicine550 First Ave, New York, NY 10016. E-mail: tomops01@nyulangone.org

PEDIATRICS (ISSN Numbers: Print, 0031-4005; Online, 1098-4275).

FINANCIAL DISCLOSURE: The authors have indicated they have no financial relationships relevant to this article to disclose.

FUNDING: No external funding.

POTENTIAL CONFLICT OF INTEREST: Dr Klass is the national medical director of Reach Out and Read (no financial compensation). Dr Mendelsohn is the principal investigator of studies of Reach Out and Read and the Video Interaction Project (no financial compensation).

COMPANION PAPER: A companion to this article can be found online at www.pediatrics.org/cgi/doi/10.1542/peds.2018-2012.

To cite: Tomopoulos S, Klass P, Mendelsohn AL. Electronic Children's Books: Promises Not Yet Fulfilled. *Pediatrics.* 2019;143(4):e20190191

COMMENTARY

Importantly, the design employed for this study was strong because it enabled comparison of parent-child interactions within dyads, potentially eliminating effects of confounding variables and supporting causal inference even with a relatively small number of study participants. These findings are consistent with limited previous studies of electronic-book enhancements in older preschool children, which also suggest that these features do not enhance supportive interactions and may work against them. The findings are also consistent with previous studies of screen time in young children, which suggest screen time interferes with verbal interactions and parent-child play[9] as well as reduces capacity for verbal and spatial learning (eg, "transfer deficit").[10] Because electronic books, unlike print books, can be "activated" by the child alone, there is a risk that solitary play with a device will replace the supportive interactions that are so important for scaffolding and early development.

This study provides evidence that electronic books as they presently exist are unlikely to result in benefits over print books for young children and are instead likely to result in barriers to interactions that are proven to be critically important for school readiness. These findings have implications for parents as they consider the reading choices they make for their children and also for clinical practice and public health policy. Regarding clinical practice, pediatricians and other child-health professionals have new data to support recommendations regarding the use of print children's books and avoiding electronics and gadgetry.[3,4] Regarding health policy, findings provide support for pediatric primary care programs, such as Reach Out and Read,[11] the Video Interaction Project,[8] and HealthySteps,[12] that can help prevent disparities in early development and school readiness through promotion of reading aloud with children's books.

There may well be a place for electronic books. Additional research is needed to understand ways to take advantage of potential benefits of this technology while still emphasizing the importance of parent-child interactions. In the meantime, pediatricians should help parents understand that enhancements often found in electronic books will not help child development as much as enhancements provided by parental interaction.

REFERENCES

1. Garner AS, Shonkoff JP; Committee on Psychosocial Aspects of Child and Family Health; Committee on Early Childhood, Adoption, and Dependent Care; Section on Developmental and Behavioral Pediatrics. Early childhood adversity, toxic stress, and the role of the pediatrician: translating developmental science into lifelong health. *Pediatrics.* 2012;129(1). Available at: www.pediatrics.org/cgi/content/full/129/1/e224
2. Munzer T, Miller A, Weeks H, Kaciroti N, Radesky J. Differences in parent-toddler interactions with electronic versus print books. *Pediatrics.* 2019;143(4): e20182012
3. High PC, Klass P; Council on Early Childhood. Literacy promotion: an essential component of primary care pediatric practice. *Pediatrics.* 2014; 134(2):404–409
4. Healey A, Mendelsohn A; Council on Early Childhood. Selecting appropriate toys for young children in the digital era. *Pediatrics.* 2019;143(1):e20183348
5. Hoff-Ginsberg E. Mother-child conversation in different social classes and communicative settings. *Child Dev.* 1991;62(4):782–796
6. Whitehurst GJ, Falco FL, Lonigan CJ, et al. Accelerating language development through picture book reading. *Dev Psychol.* 1988;24(4): 552–559
7. Mol SE, Bus AG, de Jong MT, Smeet DJ. Added value of dialogic parent–child book readings: a meta-analysis. *Early Educ Dev.* 2008;19(1):7–26
8. Mendelsohn AL, Cates CB, Weisleder A, et al. Reading aloud, play, and social-emotional development. *Pediatrics.* 2018;141(5):e20173393
9. Council on Communications and Media. Media and young minds. *Pediatrics.* 2016;138(5):e20162591
10. Barr R. Memory constraints on infant learning from picture books, television, and touchscreens. *Child Dev Perspect.* 2013;7(4):205–210
11. Klass P, Dreyer BP, Mendelsohn AL. Reach out and read: literacy promotion in pediatric primary care. *Adv Pediatr.* 2009;56:11–27
12. Minkovitz CS, Strobino D, Mistry KB, et al. Healthy steps for young children: sustained results at 5.5 years. *Pediatrics.* 2007;120(3). Available at: www.pediatrics.org/cgi/content/full/120/3/e658

Parent Verbalizations and Toddler Responses With Touchscreen Tablet Nursery Rhyme Apps

Tiffany G. Munzer, MD,[a] Alison L. Miller, PhD,[b] Samantha Yeo, BA,[a] Yujie Wang, MS,[a] Harlan McCaffery, MS,[a] Niko Kaciroti, PhD,[a,c] Jenny Radesky, MD[a]

abstract

OBJECTIVES: In some studies, parents and toddlers verbalize less when engaging with a tablet versus a print book. More needs to be known regarding child contributions to specific parent verbalizations. We examined parent-toddler contingent interactions with tablet applications versus print books, as well as moderators of these associations.

METHODS: We conducted a laboratory-based, within-subjects counterbalanced study of 72 parent-toddler dyads engaging with a nursery rhyme application (with enhanced + autonarration [E+A] and enhanced formats) and print book. We coded parent verbalizations (eg, dialogic, nondialogic) and proportions of child responses to these in 5-second epochs. Poisson regressions were used to analyze within-subjects variance by tablet or print format. We tested effect modification by child emotion regulation and home media practices.

RESULTS: Children responded more to parent overall (print 0.38; E+A 0.31, $P = .04$; enhanced 0.11, $P = .01$), dialogic (print 0.21; E+A 0.13, $P = .04$; enhanced 0.1, $P = .02$), and nondialogic (print 0.45; E+A 0.27, $P < .001$; enhanced 0.32, $P < .001$) verbalizations during print book versus tablet. Stronger child emotion regulation, greater frequency of co-viewing, and instructive practices moderated associations such that differences between conditions were no longer significant for some parent verbalizations and child responses.

CONCLUSIONS: Parent-toddler reciprocal verbal interactions occurred less frequently with tablet versus print book use. Child emotion regulation and parent home media practices moderated some of these associations. Pediatricians may wish to promote co-viewing and instructive media practices but may also consider that child emotion regulation may determine response to interactive tablet design.

Full article can be found online at www.pediatrics.org/cgi/doi/10.1542/peds.2021-049964

[a]Department of Pediatrics, Medical School and [b]Departments of Health Behavior and Health Education and [c]Biostatistics, School of Public Health, University of Michigan, Ann Arbor, Michigan

Dr Munzer drafted the initial manuscript, created the analysis plan, and reviewed and revised the manuscript; Dr Miller conceptualized and designed the study and reviewed and revised the manuscript; Ms Yeo recruited participants, developed standardized operating procedures, collected participant data, conducted data management, and reviewed and revised the manuscript; Ms Wang conducted the data management and processing and data analyses and reviewed and revised the manuscript; Mr McCaffery conducted the moderation data analyses and reviewed and revised the manuscript; Dr Kaciroti created the data analysis plan and conducted data analysis and reviewed and revised the manuscript; Dr Radesky conceptualized and designed the study, coordinated and supervised data collection, and reviewed and revised the manuscript; and all authors approved the final manuscript as submitted and agree to be accountable for all aspects of the work.

DOI: https://doi.org/10.1542/peds.2021-049964

Accepted for publication Jul 20, 2021

WHAT'S KNOWN ON THIS SUBJECT: Parent-toddler verbalizations and nonverbal indicators of social reciprocity are diminished when using some tablet applications compared with print books. No studies have examined toddler responses to specific types of parent verbalizations, and none have examined moderators of such interactions.

WHAT THIS STUDY ADDS: Toddlers exhibited lower responses to all parent verbalizations when using tablet devices compared with print books. Child emotion regulation difficulties and parent home media practices moderated associations between certain types of child responses and parent verbalizations during tablet use.

To cite: Munzer TG, Miller AL, Yeo S, et al. Parent Verbalizations and Toddler Responses With Touchscreen Tablet Nursery Rhyme Apps. *Pediatrics.* 2021;148(6):e2021049964

ARTICLE

Digital media use makes up a growing share of young children's daily activities.[1,2] More than 98% of families of young children (0–8 years old) own a mobile or tablet device,[2–4] and 2- to 4-year-olds spend on average >2 hours per day using digital media.[1,2] When toddler-aged children are using a tablet device, interactions with a responsive adult, otherwise known as joint media engagement,[5–8] can help facilitate their translation of information from the tablet into the real world.[8,9] Joint media engagement goes above and beyond the simple presence of a caregiver, with elements that include parent verbal input, child responses and/or conversational reciprocity, joint attention (both parent and child attending to the device), and parent emotional responsiveness.[10,11]

High-quality electronic book design may promote joint media engagement and emerging literacy skills in toddlers, preschool-aged children, and kindergarteners.[12–15] For example, when a book character provides dialogic reading prompts (eg, asking open-ended questions), parents exhibited more dialogic reading behaviors,[14] which has been shown to increase child responses or conversational reciprocity.[16,17] However, most commercially available electronic books and applications (apps) lack these high-quality interactive enhancements[18] and instead contain extraneous animations and advertisements that can distract young viewers.[19]

Indeed, authors of previous work have examined parent-child interactions with commercially available narrative electronic books, noting variable findings depending on the enhancements included in the electronic books.[13,20–22] In our previous work, parents exhibited fewer dialogic and total verbalizations but more format-related verbalizations (eg, comments such as "swipe the screen," "tap the picture") with a commercially available electronic tablet book compared with a print book,[23,24] and children showed lower nonverbal social reciprocity when using electronic books.[24] We did not examine toddlers' responses (eg, building on parent statements, answering questions, or acknowledging their parents) to specific types of parent verbal statements. However, different types of parent verbalizations elicit different toddler responses,[16,17] and both the parent verbalizations and child responses are 2 important aspects of joint media engagement.[11] The authors of one previous study examined toddler responses to parent verbalizations with an electronic book app containing no distracting interactive hot spots.[13] Yet most commercially available apps contain a high quantity of such extraneous design features, which may make it harder for a parent to verbally engage and for a young child to hear or notice parents' verbalizations and respond reciprocally.[25,26] To our knowledge, there have been no studies on child responses to different types of parent verbalizations (eg, dialogic, nondialogic, and format related) during use of popular apps with a high quantity of hot spots and interactivity.[18,27]

Furthermore, characteristics of the child or parent home digital media practices have not been examined in previous studies, which may shape interactions with a tablet. Yet there is a high degree of variability in how dyads engage with tablet devices.[25] For instance, children with emotion regulation difficulties may use screen media for greater durations and rely on the device as a soothing tool, which may make joint engagement more challenging. Regarding home media practices, parents' previous experiences of joint media engagement (eg, co-viewing and instruction) may also modify interactions with a tablet. Identifying moderators of parent-child interactions with the tablet may help tailor specific guidance for families.

Therefore, in this study, we aim to examine these gaps. We hypothesize that when toddlers and parents are engaging with 2 tablet apps (enhanced + autonarration [E+A] and enhanced formats) compared with a print book, (1) parents' verbalizations toward toddlers occur with lower frequency for each type of parent verbalization, with the exception of format verbalizations; (2) toddler response (verbal and nonverbal) toward parents is lower for all types of parent verbalizations; and (3) child emotion regulation difficulties (eg, negative affect, tantrum behaviors) and parent home digital media practices moderate associations with parent-child verbalizations.

METHODS

Participants

We recruited 72 parent-toddler dyads from the University of Michigan online research registry (UMHealthresearch.org), social media (eg, Facebook), and community-based settings (eg, pediatric offices, child care). Inclusion criteria were as follows: (1) child aged 24 to 36 months, (2) child without developmental delay or a serious medical condition, (3) parent able to read English sufficiently to provide consent, (4) parent the legal or physical custodial guardian, and (5) parent and child with no uncorrected hearing or vision impairments.

Procedure

This study was approved by the University of Michigan Institutional Review Board and completed in November 2018 to May 2019.

Parents provided written informed consent during the study visit. The laboratory approximated a living room, with couches, 3 books in separate boxes (2 tablets containing 1 app each, 1 print book) placed out of children's reach, a 1-way-mirror, and video cameras.

Participants first completed 5-minute video-recorded free play with nondigital toys, followed by a counterbalanced, preassigned, randomly ordered reading activity using an E+A tablet app, enhanced tablet app, and print book (with 3 different book titles). Parents received instructions to complete each activity with their toddler sequentially as prompted for 3 minutes each.

Book Formats

Three Fisher Price nursery rhyme apps were chosen because of their popularity (each app has been downloaded >1 000 000 times in the Google Play Store) and use of design elements that are widely prevalent in the children's app store. We chose nursery rhyme apps because they naturally elicit turn-taking (eg, a child completing a stanza the parent started) and gesturing compared with other toddler-directed apps. Apps were configurable in 2 settings: E+A and enhanced. Enhanced tablet app capabilities allowed for swiping to turn pages and allowed for hot spots (eg, tapping a frog resulted in the appearance of white stars with a sound effect, the nature of which was often extraneous to the nursery rhymes), in addition to the nursery rhyme instrumentation playing when swiping between pages. E+A apps had the same capabilities as the enhanced tablet, with the addition of an automatic-play sing-along when swiping between pages. For the print condition, we created a softcover print book by printing and binding high-resolution screen shots from each app page, including the nursery rhyme text. Print books were softcover and scaled to 19.1 × 11.4 cm (height × width). Apps were preloaded on a 25.4-cm Samsung Galaxy tablet. The interactive portions covered ~20.3 × 11.4 cm of the tablet screen. App 1 contained *The Itsy, Bitsy Spider* and *One, Two, Buckle My Shoe*; app 2 contained *Row, Row, Row Your Boat* and *The Animal Fair*; app 3 contained *Hickory Dickory Dock* and *Pat-a-Cake*.

Survey Measures

Parents completed surveys regarding constructs to be used as covariates and/or moderators in statistical models, including demographic information (parent's age, sex, educational attainment, household income, race and ethnicity, relationship to child, and marital status; child's age, sex, and race and ethnicity) and standardized questionnaires.

Standardized questions were used to assess frequency of home child media use (including tablet, smartphone, and electronic book usage and book reading) and parental mediation strategies (co-viewing, instructive).[28] The co-viewing subscale was used to assess the frequency with which parents watched digital media with their children; the instructive subscale was used to assess the frequency with which parents taught or explained content to children. Each subscale included 5 items rated on a 5-point Likert scale (5 = high mediation) that were then summed (Cronbach α co-viewing = 0.77, instructive = 0.87).

Toddler Emotion Regulation

Toddler emotion regulation was measured 2 ways. One included the 12-item negative affect subscale of the Early Childhood Behavioral Questionnaire Very Short Form (ECBQ), a validated, reliable[29] parent-report questionnaire of toddler temperament. Items were rated on a scale of 1 to 7 (1 = never, 7 = always) and averaged, with higher values indicating more negative affect (Cronbach α = 0.67). The second measure was an observational measure of toddler tantrums, coded in the period of time when a parent returned the tablet or book, with 0 indicating no tantrum, and 1 indicating verbal complaint, crying, or frustration (intraclass correlation = 0.88–0.96; multiple measurements due to 3 coders).[30]

Observed Parent-Toddler Exchanges (Parent Verbalizations, Toddler Conversational Reciprocity)

Because parent verbalizations elicit different child responses, the following parent verbalization categories were coded on the basis of previous work[17,21,23,31] in 5-second epochs: dialogic, nondialogic, repeats nursery rhyme, format related, off task, and behavioral management (Table 1). Codes were not mutually exclusive. Because toddlers may communicate nonverbally as well, child responses to each of these parent verbalizations were coded as response (either verbal or nonverbal) or no response (ignores parent). Child response to each type of parent verbalization category was calculated as a proportion of times children responded to their parents. Three undergraduate students blinded to the hypothesis coded to reliability, with Cohen's κ of at least 0.70 for each code (20% of videos were double-coded to ensure no coder drift).

Analysis

We conducted Poisson regressions using Proc Genmod, comparing each behavioral outcome by book format (print, enhanced, E+A). Given occasional variation in reading duration, total elapsed time was included as a covariate. All models included a repeated-measures

TABLE 1 Coding Definitions and Examples of Parent Verbalizations

	Definition	Examples	Cohen's κ Parent	Cohen's κ Child
Reads book	Parent reads book	"We went to the animal fair."	0.82	n/a
Dialogic	Dialogic reading techniques often prompt a child to expand and elaborate on concepts related to the story. These were defined as follows: parent asks open-ended question, expands on an idea the child has, repeats what the child says, or relates the story content to the child's experience	"What's happening here?" "What did they do next?" "What did you think about that?" "Remember when we went to the zoo and saw an animal?"	0.74	0.69
Nondialogic	Verbalizations that are related to story content but have not been previously shown to elicit child engagement to the degree of dialogic reading; these included the following: parent labels, asks a simple question requiring only a name or label, makes a pointing request or attention prompt, or askes the child to fill in the word	"What is that?" Parent: "The itsy bitsy . . . " child: "Spider."	0.78	0.72
Nursery rhyme	Parent repeats nursery rhyme, not reading	"The itsy bitsy spider went up the water spout."	0.84	0.79
Format related	Verbalizations that are related to the book format; parent comments, asks a question, or adds a directive on an aspect of the print or tablet interface	"Great job, you're turning the page!" "Can I hold the tablet/book?" "You can push the button here."	0.77	0.72
Off task	These are unrelated to book content or book format and include all other parent verbalizations that are not categorized	"We are going to the store after this."	0.80	0.72
Behavior management	Verbalizations in which the parent appears to be trying to redirect the child or manage the child's behavior	Child getting off the couch; parent says, "Get back here!" "You can have your goldfish later."	0.74	0.70

Child response was coded for each of these types of parent verbalizations as present (1), including a verbal response or a nonverbal acknowledgment, or absent (0). n/a, not applicable.

statement to allow for within-subjects comparison of behavioral outcomes by book format, and order effects were accounted for. Covariates in final models with $P < .05$ were included to improve model fit (eg, income-to-needs ratio, marital status, etc). Race and ethnicity was included as a potential covariate if $P < .05$ because of previous work identifying systemic inequities in digital media access (eg, lack of reliable Wi-Fi) for Black and Latinx populations.[32] We tested effect modification by creating interaction terms between 2 measures of child emotion regulation difficulties (ECBQ negative affect, tantrums) and 2 types of parent home digital media practices (co-viewing, instructive) and parent verbalizations and child responses with tablet or book use. All analyses were completed in SAS 9.4 (SAS Institute, Inc, Cary, NC).

RESULTS

As shown in Table 2, children were 30.2 months of age, and parents were 33.0 years of age. Of the parents, 93% were mothers, 69% had a 4-year college degree or greater, and 89% were married. Of the children, 40% were boys and 74% were White non-Hispanic.

Overall, parents had fewer total verbalizations (excluding reading) during tablet use in either tablet condition compared with print book use (E+A mean 27.16 [SD = 1.47] versus print mean 35.95 [SD = 1.17], $P < .001$; enhanced mean 30.46 [SD = 1.35] versus print mean 35.95 [SD = 1.17], $P < .001$; enhanced versus E+A $P < .001$). As shown in Fig 1, parents read the app or book more in the enhanced tablet and print book compared with the E+A tablet (enhanced 8.84 [0.54] versus print 8.49 [0.55], $P = .58$; E+A 4.19 [0.43] versus print 8.49 [0.55], $P < .001$; enhanced versus E+A $P = .58$). Use of both tablet formats resulted in fewer parent dialogic verbalizations compared with print book use (E+A 1.74 [0.19] versus print 3.65 [0.43], $P < .001$; enhanced 1.62 [0.19] versus print 3.65 [0.43], $P < .001$; enhanced versus E+A $P = .52$). There were fewer nondialogic verbalizations during use of both tablet formats compared with print book use (E+A 11.78 [0.68] versus print 17.43 [0.81], $P < .001$; enhanced 11.80 [0.67] versus print 17.43 [0.81], $P < .001$; enhanced versus E+A $P = .97$). Parents repeated the nursery rhyme with

TABLE 2 Participant Characteristics

Study Sample	N = 72
Child age, mo, mean (SD)	30.2 (3.8)
Parent age, y, mean (SD)	33.0 (4.3)
Parent relationship to child, n (%)	
Mother	67 (93)
Father	5 (7)
Child sex, n (%)	
Male	29 (40)
Female	43 (60)
Child race and ethnicity, n (%)	
White, non-Hispanic	53 (74)
Black, Hispanic, Asian, Pacific Islander, or biracial	19 (26)
Parent education, n (%)	
High school or GED	4 (6)
Some college courses	12 (17)
2-y college degree	6 (8)
4-y college degree	24 (33)
>4-y college degree	26 (36)
Parent marital status, n (%)	
Single	2 (3)
Married	62 (86)
In a committed relationship	4 (6)
Separated or divorced	4 (6)
ECBQ negative affect score, mean (SD)	2.9 (0.6)
No. children with presence of tantrums, n (%)	20 (28)
Child has actively used smartphone, n (%)	66 (92)
Child has actively used iPad or tablet, n (%)	55 (76)
Time child has spent using iPad, tablet, or smartphone on the most typical weekday, n (%)	
Not used or never	36 (51)
<30 min	18 (25)
30 min to 1 h	6 (9)
1–2 h	9 (13)
2–3 h	1 (1)
3–4 h	1 (1)
Time child has spent reading with adult on the most typical weekday	
Not used or never	6 (8)
<30 min	22 (31)
30 min to 1 h	33 (46)
1–2 h	9 (13)
3–4 h	1 (1)
Co-viewing, mean (SD)	14.6 (3.0)
Instructive, mean (SD)	15.5 (3.5)

GED, general equivalency diploma.

lower frequency when using the E+A tablet format compared with the enhanced tablet and print formats but had more format-related verbalizations, fewer off-task verbalizations, and fewer behavioral comments when using both tablet formats compared with the print format.

Overall, child conversational response was lower for parent verbalizations during tablet use in either tablet condition compared with print book use (E+A proportion 0.31 [SD = 0.02] versus print proportion 0.38 [SD = 0.02], P = .004; enhanced proportion 0.30 [0.02] versus print proportion 0.38 [SD = 0.02], P < .001; enhanced versus E+A P = .039). Figure 2 reveals the proportion of child responses to each type of parent verbalization. Children responded to fewer dialogic verbalizations during tablet use in either tablet condition compared with print book use (E+A 0.13 [0.03] versus print 0.21 [0.03], P = .04; enhanced 0.11 [0.03] versus print 0.21 [0.03], P = .02; enhanced versus E+A P = .58). Children responded to fewer parent nondialogic verbalizations during tablet use in either tablet condition compared with print book use (E+A 0.27 [0.02] versus print 0.45 [0.03], P < .001; enhanced 0.32 [0.03] versus print 0.45 [0.03], P < .001; enhanced versus E+A P = .04). Children responded to fewer parent nursery rhyme verbalizations during tablet use in either tablet condition compared with print book use (E+A 0.12 [0.03] versus print 0.24 [0.04], P = .01; enhanced 0.07 [0.02] versus print 0.24 [0.04], P < .001; enhanced versus E+A P = .08). However, children responded to more parent format-related verbalizations during tablet use in either tablet condition compared with print book use (E+A 0.51 [0.04] versus print 0.27 [0.07], P = .01; enhanced 0.53 [0.04] versus print 0.27 [0.07], P = .01; enhanced versus E+A P = .54). There were no differences in child responses to parent off-task or behavioral verbalizations across all 3 conditions.

As shown in the Fig 3 moderation analyses, child emotion regulation characteristics moderated some parent verbalizations and child responses. ECBQ negative affect moderated child response to parent nursery rhyme verbalizations (P = .03) such that children with high negative affect responded to their parents more when using the print book versus the E+A tablet; this was no different for children with low negative affect. Child tantrums moderated parent nondialogic verbalizations (P = .004) such that parent nondialogic verbalizations were greater in the print book condition versus the E+A tablet condition for children without tantrums, and this was no different for children with tantrums.

Parent home digital media practices moderated some parent

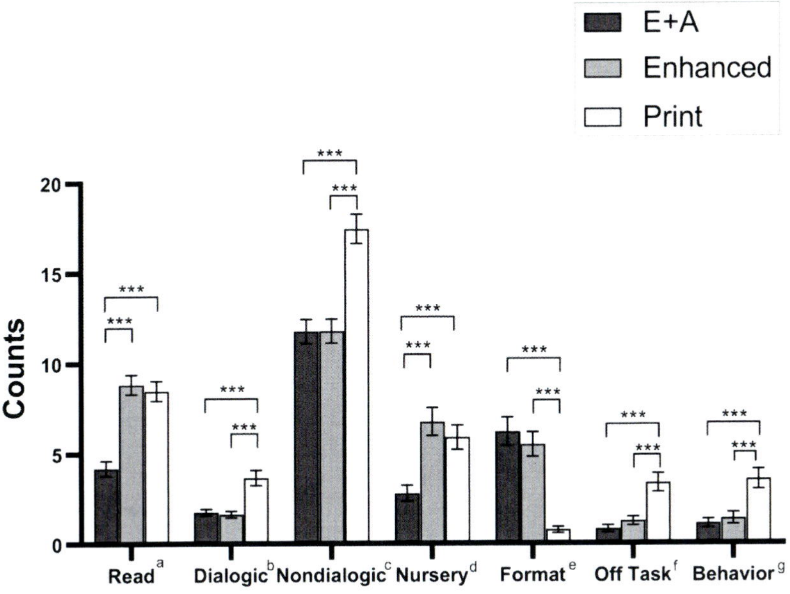

FIGURE 1
Parent verbalization counts (average verbalizations for parents by each type of book format). Footnotes represent covariates included in models. [a] Book title. [b] Parenting self-efficacy and book title. [c] Parenting self-efficacy, child race and ethnicity, and parent race and ethnicity. [d] Book title and child race and ethnicity. [e] Marital status. [f] ITN and marital status. [g] No additional covariates. *** $P < .001$. ITN, income-to-needs ratio.

verbalizations and child responses. Co-viewing moderated the child response to parent nursery rhyme verbalizations during use of the E+A tablet ($P = .003$) such that children exposed to greater co-viewing responded more to their parents during use of the E+A tablet compared with children exposed to lower co-viewing. Instructive media practices moderated parent nursery rhyme verbalizations during use of the E+A tablet ($P = .006$) such that parent nursery rhyme verbalizations were lower during use of the E+A tablet, resulting in greater differences between E+A tablet and print book use in those with low instruction compared with those with high instruction. Instructive media practices moderated parent dialogic verbalizations during use of the enhanced tablet ($P = .01$) such that dialogic verbalizations were higher during print book use, resulting in a greater difference between enhanced tablet and print book use for children exposed to greater instruction compared with lower instruction. Instructive media practices moderated child response to nursery rhyme verbalizations during use of the enhanced tablet ($P = .04$) such that children with high instruction responded similarly to their parents when using print and tablet formats, and those with low instruction responded more to their parents when using a print book compared with either tablet format.

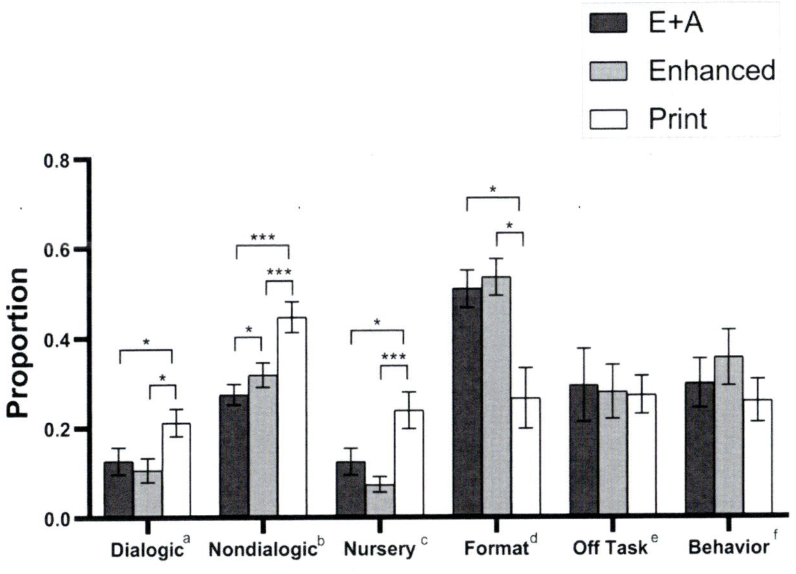

FIGURE 2
Child response, in proportions, to each parent verbalization type. Footnotes represent covariates included in models. [a] Child age and book title. [b] Child age and marital status [c] Child sex. [d] Parent age and book title. [e] Child age, parenting self-efficacy, and ITN. [f] Child age and marital status. * $P < .05$; *** $P < .001$. ITN, income-to-needs ratio.

DISCUSSION

Parent-child interactions are central correlates of future child developmental outcomes (language, peer relationships, academic achievement),[33–37] which are shaped by several aspects of the environment,[38,39] including digital media.[26,40] We found that toddler responses to parent verbalizations (a central aspect of parent-child conversational reciprocity) was lower during use of both E+A and enhanced tablet nursery rhyme apps compared with a print book use. Not only were parent verbalizations toward toddlers less frequent in the tablet conditions but also a majority

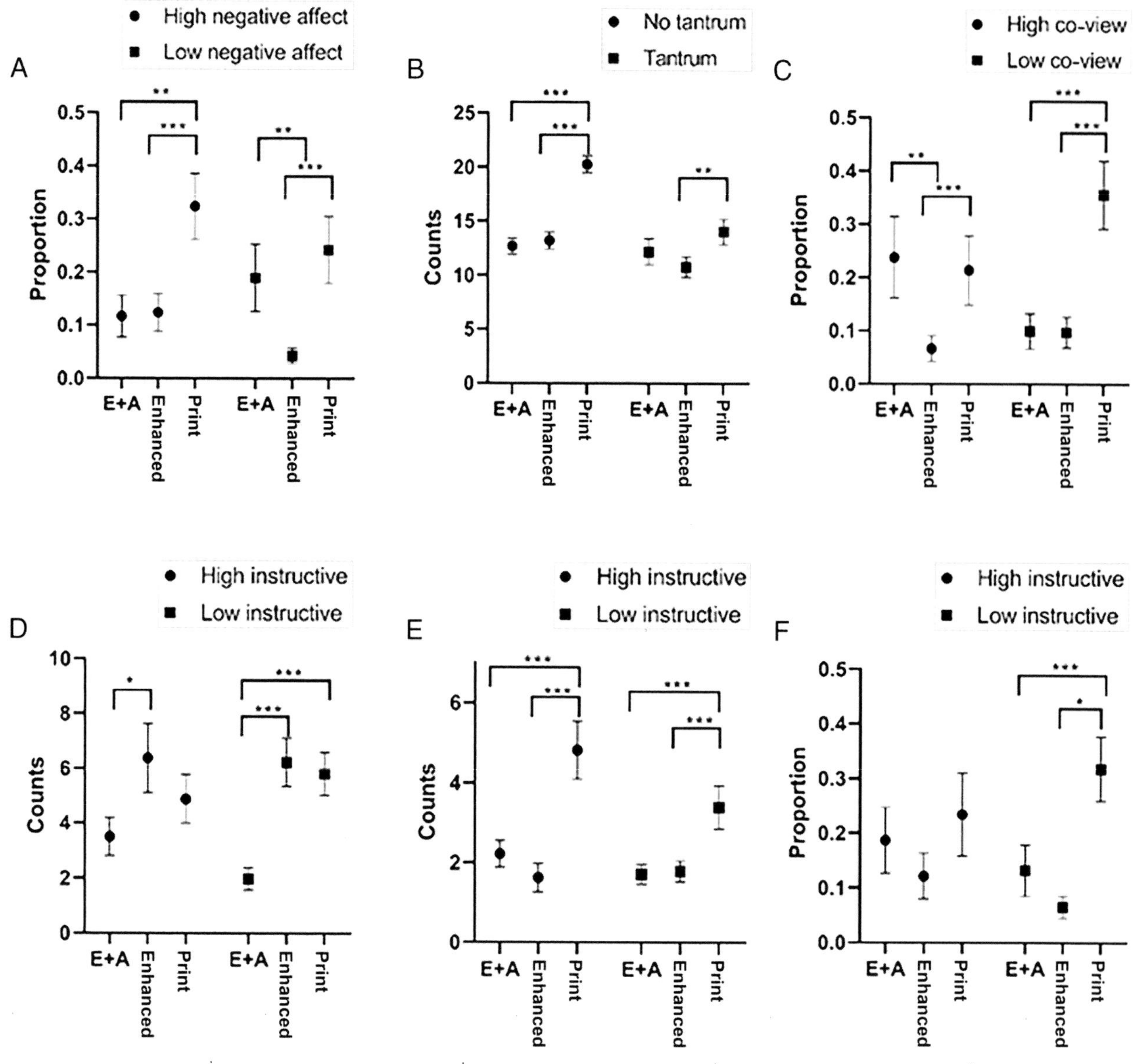

FIGURE 3
Effect modification results after stratifying for child individual characteristics (ECBQ negative affect, presence of tantrums) and home digital media practices (co-viewing, instructive). A, Child nursery rhyme. B, Parent nondialogic. C, Child nursery rhyme. D, Parent nursery rhyme. E, Parent dialogic. F, Child nursery rhyme. * $P < .05$; ** $P < .01$; *** $P < .001$.

of these verbalizations were ignored by toddlers and to a more substantial degree when using tablets compared with a print book.

Parent verbalization results were similar to those in our previous study (in which we used an app with less interactivity),[23] revealing fewer dialogic, nondialogic, and overall verbalizations from parents, suggesting that previous findings generalize to apps with stronger visual features and distractions. It is possible that the app we chose with common nursery rhymes may not promote dialogic reading practices to the same degree as more narrative books, and perhaps the E+A app might not have allowed sufficient time for parents to verbalize and children to respond because of autonarration. Our work is similar to previous findings among preschool-aged children reading electronic books that include interactive hot spots[20–22] but differs from one study that found similar parent verbalizations with an electronic book without hot spots[13] and print books. This suggests that such interactive hot spots may impede parents' optimal ability to verbally engage with their children. Differing from our previous work,[23] we found greater parent behavioral verbalizations during use of the print book compared with the tablet apps.

Such interactive hot spots and tablet design features may also come at the expense of children's response to parents' verbalizations and parent-child conversational reciprocity. In this experimental paradigm, toddlers responded to their parents less when using the tablet, even when the parents were engaging in dialogic techniques. Nevertheless, diminished child responsivity in both tablet conditions was noted overall and across almost each parent verbalization category (dialogic, nondialogic, and nursery rhyme). Because parent-child interactional patterns are transactional in nature (eg, parents adjust their approach depending on their children's responses),[41] we surmise that low child response to parents could mean that over time, parents may minimize the quantity of parent verbalizations when engaging with tablet devices. This may reflect differences in how parents tailored their verbalizations to their children in our results. For instance, in the enhanced and E+A conditions, children responded to more format-related verbalizations compared with the print condition, which may have led parents to exhibit greater format-related verbalizations.

Child emotion regulation difficulties moderated associations between child response to nursery rhymes and parent nondialogic verbalizations. This suggests that (1) children with emotion regulation difficulties may struggle with responding to parent verbalizations while engaging with tablet devices and (2) their parents may adjust their verbalizations as a result. In contrast, home media practices, such as co-viewing and instruction, may also promote certain types of parent verbalizations and children's responses. Households engaging in co-viewing and instructive practices may promote more conversational reciprocity when using a tablet compared with households engaging in such practices less frequently because the dyad may be used to interacting in this manner.

Fluent, connected, and reciprocal conversation in the toddler years has been associated with improved expressive language development in preschool[42] and greater social competence in future peer interactions and academic achievement into adolescence.[43] Such interactions from both toddlers and parents are occurring with lower frequency with tablet use compared with print book use. Limitations of this study included a sample slightly more White and college educated than the general population, which may limit the study generalizability to other populations. Strengths include use of a tablet app with common design features, within-subjects approach, and observational coding of parent and child behavior. Next steps might include sequential analysis of parent-toddler conversational reciprocity (and conversational turn-taking), assessing the parent and toddler emotional experience when co-viewing, and replicating this study in a more racially and ethnically diverse sample.

CONCLUSIONS

Tablets and mobile devices are prominent fixtures in modern family life, and app design features can impede children's responses despite parent's efforts to engage their children in developmentally enriching conversation. Software designers could consider limiting extraneous enhancements for young children and incorporating feedback from trained early childhood specialists. Pediatric providers should continue recommending engagement in co-viewing and instructive home media practices when possible (eg, by asking open-ended questions) and focus on ways to incorporate dialogic practices when possible. Lastly, pediatric providers may also wish to note that some children have varying responses to digital media and that children with emotion regulation challenges may have more difficulties interacting with a tablet device, even in the context of joint media engagement.

ABBREVIATIONS

E+A: enhanced + autonarration
ECBQ: Early Childhood Behavioral Questionnaire Very Short Form

Address correspondence to Tiffany G. Munzer, MD, University of Michigan, 300 N Ingalls St, 1027NW, Ann Arbor, MI 48109-5406. E-mail: chungti@med.umich.edu

PEDIATRICS (ISSN Numbers: Print, 0031-4005; Online, 1098-4275).

FINANCIAL DISCLOSURE: Dr Radesky is paid to write articles for the PBS Parents Web site and is on the board of directors of and consults for Melissa & Doug, LLC; the other authors have indicated they have no financial relationships relevant to this article to disclose.

FUNDING: Funded by the *Eunice Kennedy Shriver* National Institute of Child Health and Development (grant 5R03HD94077), which made it possible to conceptualize, implement, collect, and analyze data and write this article. Funded by the National Institutes of Health (NIH).

POTENTIAL CONFLICT OF INTEREST: Dr Radesky is paid to write articles for the PBS Parents Web site and is on the board of directors of and consults for Melissa & Doug, LLC; the other authors have indicated they have no potential conflicts of interest to disclose.

REFERENCES

1. Radesky JS, Weeks HM, Ball R, et al. Young children's use of smartphones and tablets. *Pediatrics.* 2020;146(1):e20193518
2. Rideout V, Robb MB. *The Common Sense Census: Media Use by Kids Age Zero to Eight.* San Francisco, CA: Common Sense Media; 2020
3. Rideout V. *The Common Sense Census: Media Use by Kids Age Zero to Eight.* San Francisco, CA: Common Sense Media; 2017
4. Kabali HK, Irigoyen MM, Nunez-Davis R, et al. Exposure and use of mobile media devices by young children. *Pediatrics.* 2015;136(6): 1044–1050
5. Choi K, Kirkorian HL. Touch or watch to learn? Toddlers' object retrieval using contingent and noncontingent video. *Psychol Sci.* 2016;27(5):726–736
6. Huber B, Meyer D, Kaufman J. Young children's contingent interactions with a touchscreen influence their memory for spatial and narrative content. *Media Psychol.* 2020;23(4):552–578
7. Kirkorian HL, Choi K, Pempek TA. Toddlers' word learning from contingent and noncontingent video on touch screens. *Child Dev.* 2016;87(2):405–413
8. Strouse GA, Troseth GL, O'Doherty KD, Saylor MM. Co-viewing supports toddlers' word learning from contingent and noncontingent video. *J Exp Child Psychol.* 2018;166:310–326
9. Sims C, Colunga E. Parent-child screen media co-viewing: influences on toddlers' word learning and retention. In: Proceedings of the Annual Meeting of the Cognitive Science Society; July 31–August 3, 2013; Berlin Germany
10. Padilla-Walker LM, Coyne SM, Booth MA, et al. Parent–child joint media engagement in infancy. *Infancy.* 2020;25(5):552–570
11. Ewin CA, Reupert AE, McLean LA, Ewin CJ. The impact of joint media engagement on parent–child interactions: a systematic review. *Hum Behav Emerg Technol.* 2021;3(2):230–254
12. Strouse GA, Ganea PA. Toddlers' word learning and transfer from electronic and print books. *J Exp Child Psychol.* 2017;156:129–142
13. Strouse GA, Ganea PA. Parent-toddler behavior and language differ when reading electronic and print picture books. *Front Psychol.* 2017;8:677
14. Troseth GL, Strouse GA, Flores I, Stuckelman ZD, Johnson CR. An enhanced eBook facilitates parent–child talk during shared reading by families of low socioeconomic status. *Early Child Res Q.* 2020;50(pt 1):45–58
15. Rvachew S, Rees K, Carolan E, Nadig A. Improving emergent literacy with school-based shared reading: paper versus ebooks. *Int J Child Comput Interact.* 2017;12:24–29
16. Arnold DS, Whitehurst GJ. Accelerating language development through picture book reading: a summary of dialogic reading and its effect. In: Dickinson DK, ed. *Bridges to Literacy: Children, Families, and Schools.* Hoboken, NJ: Blackwell Publishing; 1994:103–128
17. Whitehurst GJ, Arnold DS, Epstein JN, Angell AL, Smith M, Fischel JE. A picture book reading intervention in day care and home for children from low-income families. *Dev Psychol.* 1994;30(5):679–689
18. Meyer M, Zosh JM, McLaren C, et al. How educational are "educational" apps for young children? App store content analysis using the Four Pillars of Learning framework [published online ahead of print February 23, 2021]. *J Child Media.* doi:10.1080/17482798.2021.1882516
19. Takacs ZK, Swart EK, Bus AG. Benefits and pitfalls of multimedia and interactive features in technology-enhanced storybooks: a meta-analysis. *Rev Educ Res.* 2015;85(4):698–739
20. Krcmar M, Cingel DP. Parent–child joint reading in traditional and electronic formats. *Media Psychol.* 2014;17(3): 262–281
21. Chiong C, Ree J, Takeuchi L, Erickson I. Comparing parent-child co-reading on print, basic, and enhanced e-book platforms: a Cooney Center QuickReport. 2012. Available at: https://joanganzcooneycenter.org/publication/quickreport-print-books-vs-e-books/. Accessed February 1, 2021
22. Parish-Morris J, Mahajan N, Hirsh-Pasek K, Golinkoff RM, Collins MF. Once upon a time: parent–child dialogue and storybook reading in the electronic era. *Mind Brain Educ.* 2013;7(3):200–211
23. Munzer TG, Miller AL, Weeks HM, Kaciroti N, Radesky J. Differences in parent-toddler interactions with electronic versus print books. *Pediatrics.* 2019;143(4):e20182012
24. Munzer TG, Miller AL, Weeks HM, Kaciroti N, Radesky J. Parent-toddler social reciprocity during reading from electronic tablets vs print books. *JAMA Pediatr.* 2019;173(11):1076–1083
25. Hiniker A, Lee B, Kientz JA, Radesky JS. Let's play!: digital and analog play between preschoolers and parents. In: Proceedings of the 2018 CHI Conference on Human Factors in Computing Systems; April 21–26, 2018; Montreal, Canada
26. Radesky JS, Kistin CJ, Zuckerman B, et al. Patterns of mobile device use by caregivers and children during meals in fast food restaurants. *Pediatrics.* 2014;133(4). Available at: www.pediatrics.org/cgi/content/full/133/4/e843
27. Hirsh-Pasek K, Zosh JM, Golinkoff RM, Gray JH, Robb MB, Kaufman J. Putting education in "educational" apps: lessons from the science of learning. *Psychol Sci Public Interest.* 2015;16(1):3–34
28. Valkenburg PM, Krcmar M, Peeters AL, Marseille NM. Developing a scale to assess three styles of television mediation: "instructive mediation," "restrictive mediation," and "social coviewing". *J Broadcast Electron Media.* 1999;43(1):52–66
29. Putnam SP, Helbig AL, Gartstein MA, Rothbart MK, Leerkes E. Development and assessment of short and very

short forms of the infant behavior questionnaire-revised. *J Pers Assess.* 2014;96(4):445–458

30. Munzer TG, Miller AL, Wang Y, Kaciroti N, Radesky J. Tablets, toddlers, and tantrums: the immediate effects of tablet device play. *Acta Paediatr.* 2021;110(1): 255–256
31. Lauricella AR, Barr R, Calvert SL. Parent–child interactions during traditional and computer storybook reading for children's comprehension: implications for electronic storybook design. *Int J Child Comput Interact.* 2014;2(1):17–25
32. Katz VS, Gonzalez C, Clark K. Digital inequality and developmental trajectories of low-income, immigrant, and minority children. *Pediatrics.* 2017;140(suppl 2): S132–S136
33. Belsky J, Fearon RM. Early attachment security, subsequent maternal sensitivity, and later child development: does continuity in development depend upon continuity of caregiving? *Attach Hum Dev.* 2002;4(3):361–387
34. Bus AG, Belsky J, van Ijzendoom MH, Crnic K. Attachment and bookreading patterns: a study of mothers, fathers, and their toddlers. *Early Child Res Q.* 1997;12(1):81–98
35. Evans CA, Porter CL. The emergence of mother-infant co-regulation during the first year: links to infants' developmental status and attachment. *Infant Behav Dev.* 2009;32(2):147–158
36. Frosch CA, Cox MJ, Goldman BD. Infant-parent attachment and parental and child behavior during parent-toddler storybook interaction. *Merrill-Palmer Q.* 2001;47(4):445–474
37. George C, Solomon J. Attachment and caregiving: the caregiving behavioral system. In: Cassidy J, Shaver PR, eds. *Handbook of Attachment: Theory, Research, and Clinical Applications.* New York, NY; The Guilford Press; 1999:649–670
38. Zuckerman B, Needlman R. 30 years of Reach Out and Read: need for a developmental perspective. *Pediatrics.* 2020;145(6):e20191958
39. Härkönen U. *The Bronfenbrenner Ecological Systems Theory of Human Development.* Scientific Articles of V International Conference. Latvia, 2001
40. Linebarger DL, Vaala SE. Screen media and language development in infants and toddlers: an ecological perspective. *Dev Rev.* 2010;30(2):176–202
41. Sameroff A. Transactional models in early social relations. *Hum Dev.* 1975;18(1–2):65–79
42. Hirsh-Pasek K, Adamson LB, Bakeman R, et al. The contribution of early communication quality to low-income children's language success. *Psychol Sci.* 2015;26(7):1071–1083
43. Gil-Olarte Márquez P, Palomera Martín R, Brackett MA. Relating emotional intelligence to social competence and academic achievement in high school students. *Psicothema.* 2006; 18(suppl):118–123